Contraception Today

*A Pocketbook for General Practitioners
and Practice Nurses
Seventh Edition*

John Guillebaud
*Emeritus Professor of
Family Planning and
Reproductive Health,
University College London
UK*

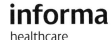

informa
healthcare

This book represents the personal opinions of John Guillebaud, based wherever possible on published and sometimes unpublished evidence. When (as is not infrequent) no epidemiological or other direct evidence is available, clinical advice herein is always as practical and realistic as possible and based, pending more data, on the author's judgement of other sources. These may include the opinions of Expert Committees and any existing Guidelines. In some instances the advice appearing in this book may even so differ appreciably from the latter, for reasons usually given in the text and (since medical knowledge and practice are continually evolving) it relates to the date of publication. Healthcare professionals must understand that they take ultimate responsibility for their patient and ensure that any clinical advice they use from this book is applicable to the specific circumstances that they encounter.

A CIP record for this book is available from the British Library.

ISBN-13: 9781841849119

Orders may be sent to: Informa Healthcare, Sheepen Place, Colchester, Essex CO3 3LP, UK
Telephone: +44 (0)20 7017 5540
Email: CSDhealthcarebooks@informa.com
Website: http://informahealthcarebooks.com/

Library of Congress Cataloging-in-Publication Data

Guillebaud, John.
    Contraception today : a pocketbook for general practitioners and practice nurses / John Guillebaud. -- 7th ed.
        p. ; cm.
    Includes bibliographical references and index.
    ISBN 978-1-84184-911-9 (pbk. : alk. paper)
    I. Title.
    [DNLM: 1. Contraceptive Agents--Handbooks. 2. Contraception--Handbooks. 3. Contraceptive Devices--Handbooks. QV 39]

    615.7′66–dc23

                                                                    2011037708

For corporate sales please contact: CorporateBooksIHC@informa.com
For foreign rights please contact: RightsIHC@informa.com
For reprint permissions please contact: PermissionsIHC@informa.com
Typeset by MPS Ltd, Delhi
Printed and bound in the United Kingdom by CPI Antony Rowe Ltd, Chippenham, Wiltshire

Statement of competing interests
The author has received payments for research projects, lectures, *ad hoc* consultancy work and related expenses from the manufacturers of contraceptive products.

Contents

Preface

... how successful we have become. We as a species together with our cows, pigs etc, we are about 97 per cent of the biomass of all vertebrate species, meaning only 3 per cent are wild species.

Mathis Wackernagel, in The Ecological Footprint, 2005

We have not inherited the earth from our grandparents, we have borrowed it from our grandchildren.

Kashmiri proverb

Family planning could bring more benefits to more people at less cost than any other single technology now available to the human race.

James Grant, UNICEF, 1992

Climate change absolutely must increase with growth in the numbers of climate changERS.

More Humanity with fewer Humans

Slogans of *Population Matters*/Optimum Population Trust

I have not seen an environmental problem that wouldn't be easier to solve with fewer people, or harder, and ultimately impossible, with ever more.

Sir David Attenborough, Patron of Population Matters

Born and reared in Burundi and Rwanda, countries whose recurrent agonies are in significant measure related to excessive population growth, I maintain that:

Human **needs** along with those of all other species with which we share the Natural World will never be sustainably met on a finite planet without more concerned, non-coercive, action on human **numbers**.

No woman on earth who at time present wishes to exercise her human right to have *the choice* to control her fertility should be denied the means to do so, by barriers produced by any agency— whether through her partner's refusal, her society's pro-natalism, misinformation (sometimes deliberate), or lack of available, affordable and accessible contraceptive supplies and services.

Isn't over-population an overseas problem? Not so, in their lifetime, every new birth in the United Kingdom will, through the inevitable effluence of his or her affluence as a consumer, harm the environment—by climate change and in numerous other ways—as much as 30, or on some criteria 200, times more than births in Burundi or Bangladesh will ever do. We cannot be proud of our record in preventing teenage conceptions, and even in 2012 in all age groups conceptions still occur too often by chance rather than by choice. So we all have a part to play in ensuring that our grandchildren receive back their 'loan' in a halfway decent and long-term sustainable state. As a small but relevant contribution to that endeavour, I welcome this opportunity to bring a new edition of this pocketbook on contraception to general practitioners and nurses in primary care. (See also www.ecotimecapsule.com.)

I write, moreover, as one who is proud to have worked in general practice, as a locum in places as diverse as Barnsley, Cambridge, Luton and South London, and hence able to appreciate some of the satisfactions and the constraints of that role.

January 2012

Acknowledgements
I wish to thank numerous friends and colleagues in the United Kingdom and abroad working in relevant specialist and general practice—too many to mention all by name. Dr Diana Mansour and Dr Anne MacGregor deserve special mention, also Toni Belfield, formerly Head of Information at the UK FPA, and Robert Peden (of the Informa Healthcare Imprint) who has guided this work through nearly all of its seven editions. I acknowledge repeated help from staff of the Clinical Effectiveness Unit of the Faculty of Sexual and Reproductive Health (FSRH) and, over many years, from senior medical and nursing staff at the Margaret Pyke Centre (MPC) and Oxford Family Planning Clinics. Finally, I am also grateful to some of our clients for the insights they have given me over the years.

John Guillebaud is Emeritus Professor of Family Planning and Reproductive Health at University College London, and Research Director at the Elliot-Smith Vasectomy Clinic, Churchill Hospital, Oxford.

Until 2002, he was Medical Director of the Margaret Pyke Centre in London, and continues as a Trustee of the Margaret Pyke Trust.

Introduction

General practitioners (GPs) and practice nurses are often best placed to offer good contraceptive advice because they already know the patient's health and family circumstances. Some practices are excellent; others provide little beyond oral contraception and devote insufficient time and skill to counselling. The 2002 Sexual Health Strategy established that primary care should always supply at least Level 1 basic contraceptive services, and should also consider supplying services at Level 2. These include all the long-acting reversible contraceptive methods (LARCs). The National Institute for Health and Clinical Excellence (NICE) Clinical Guideline No. 30 (www.nice.org.uk, 2005, to be updated in 2012) drew attention to the many contraceptive (and sometimes non-contraceptive) advantages of these, comprising injectables, implants, the latest copper-banded intrauterine devices (IUDs) and the levonorgestrel intrauterine system (LNG-IUS). If not supplied on site, practices should have referral arrangements in place for the LARCs, agreed to be within 24 hours for copper IUDs as emergency contraception; and also when appropriate for Level 3 services such as male and female sterilization, and medical or surgical abortion.

Iatrogenic ('doctor-caused') pregnancies are a reality. They result from avoidable errors or omissions on the part of service providers, especially the omission of sufficient time for the consultation.

Women choosing their first-ever 'medical' contraceptive need more than the usual 10 minutes available in most surgeries. Indeed, it is recommended that 'at least 20 minutes should be allocated to a practitioner or clinical team (e.g. nurse + doctor) for … a new consultation … a new contraceptive method' (Service standards on workload in sexual and reproductive health (SRH), 2009; www.fsrh.org/pdfs/ServiceStandardsforWorkload0509.pdf).

Writing as 'an ex-GP', 20 minutes is obviously daunting yet not unreasonable, when one considers the ground to be covered, say for a first-time Pill-user (see pp. 61–2). An arrangement that works well in some practices is to offer routinely a second 10 to 15 minute consultation within the same week, either at the end of a surgery or with the practice nurse.

Much of this work can—indeed should—be the responsibility of practice nurses fully trained in family planning, usually with a gain rather than a loss in standards. Practice is changing fast, with more use of patient group directions and more nurse practitioners who are prescribers, some of whom with additional training insert intrauterine and subdermal contraceptives. A good 'mainstream' practice nurse may perform the following delegated functions appropriately:

- Taking sexual and medical histories, discussing choices [using UK Family Planning Association (fpa) leaflets]
- Pill teaching
- Pill issuing/reissuing and emergency Pill issuing—given fully agreed and audited patient group directions
- Pill monitoring, including migraine assessment and blood pressure (BP)
- Giving contraceptive injections: depot medroxyprogesterone acetate (DMPA; Depo-Provera™)
- IUD and IUS checking, including eliciting cervical excitation tenderness
- Cervical smear taking

Formal training through the FSRH* is ideal for doctors and should include both theoretical and 'apprenticeship' training, as well as

*In the United Kingdom, the Faculty of Sexual and Reproductive Healthcare (FSRH) offers training, through a combination of e-learning available at its website www.fsrh.org, a theoretical assessment day and on-site training arranged regionally, leading to a Diploma (DFSRH) or Membership (MFSRH), as well as Letters of Competence (LOC) in intrauterine techniques, subdermal implants and medical education. Since 2002, nurses and associate practitioners working in reproductive health have been eligible to become Associates of the Faculty.

The Institute of Psychosexual Medicine (www.ipm.org.uk) and the College for Sexual and Relationship Therapy (www.cosrt.org.uk) also offer relevant training courses and seminars.

discussion of the often complex psychosexual and emotional factors involved in the use of contraception. All clinicians should be sensitive to hidden signals in this area.

Doctors or nurses should back their counselling with good literature. Although some manufacturers have improved their patient information leaflets (PILs), the latest fpa leaflets are user friendly, accurate and comprehensive. The one called *Your Guide to Contraception* tabulates all the important methods, both reversible and permanent, and is ideal for reading in the waiting room before counselling. The leaflets on individual methods can be downloaded from the fpa website in up-to-date versions and should be given with advice to 'read, and keep long term for further reference'. Together with accurate contemporary records, these leaflets provide strong medicolegal backup for practitioners who may be asked to justify their actions in the event of litigation. They are an essential supplement to—but by no means a replacement for—time spent with the health care practitioner.

CHOICE OF METHOD

Most women who seek contraception are healthy and young, and present fewer problems than those over 35, teenagers and those with intercurrent disease. There is a tendency for sterilization procedures to be demanded at too early an age. This is partly because the Pill is too often seen as synonymous with contraception, and we as providers have not been informing women about the many new or improved reversible alternatives, about which there is still much mythology and ignorance. See Figure 1: the methods at bottom left are known collectively as the LARCs— the LNG-IUS, the banded copper IUDs, injectables and the latest implants. All of these can be seen as reversible sterilization, since essentially their efficacy is truly 'in the same ballpark' as female sterilization.

THE YOUNG

I am opposed to 'sex education'! This is because I support—as we all should—sex *and relationships* education (SRE). When seeking advice on sex, relationships, contraception, pregnancy and parenthood, young people are entitled to accessible,

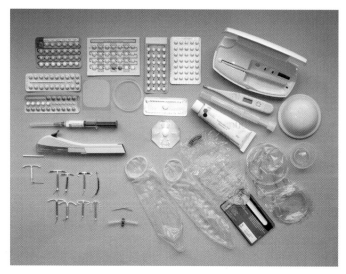

Figure 1
The choice of methods in the United Kingdom (2012). Source: Courtesy of Dr Anne MacGregor.

confidential, non-judgemental and unbiased support and guidance, recognizing the diversity of their cultural and faith traditions. We should listen to their views and respect their opinions and choices. Valid choices include waiting ('saving sex') as well as having (safer and contracepted) sex.

It is not a good idea to have sex only because:
- someone else wants you to
- someone says they'll leave you if you don't
- all your friends say they are doing it
- you feel too scared to say 'no'
- OR: when it just doesn't seem right to you (with this person or now)

Slightly altered from www.likeitis.org

However, as they may often 'get away with it' in one or more cycles, all too often the young do not seek advice until they have already conceived. Easier access to emergency contraception is an obvious priority. But education *for both genders* must promote (as in the Netherlands) the societal norm that, unless conception is planned, sex may be a feature of a good relationship only when and if adequate contraception exists. In this age group, we still await improved first-line more 'forgettable' methods in which (in contrast to the Pill) non-pregnancy is the default state. We already do have the LARCs; injectables and implants (best used in this order, see pp. 110,112) are usually preferable to copper IUDs although these are only relatively contraindicated (WHO 2, usually p. 138) and that option should surely be offered as emergency contraception more often than it is (p. 146).

The LNG-IUS may also be appropriate for some young people, though not post-coitally (p. 136).

Confidentiality and related issues
- Is your practice SRH service's confidentiality policy explicit, *and* implicit: i.e. does it *feel* cast-iron to her/him?
- Does the young person (<16 *or not*) understand her/his rights— '*including the right not to have or delay having sex* ... and how to negotiate safer sex?'
- Might there be *abuse* or *coercion*? Check girl's partner's age— and hers (is she really not under 13?).
- If it therefore becomes necessary for others or other agencies to become involved, always inform the young person.
- All SRH services 'should have a named person identified as the local lead for child protection'.
- 'First intercourse is often associated with regret, feeling pressured and alcohol consumption.'

From FSRH Guidance *Contraceptive Choices for Young People*, March 2010

For young people under 16 years of age, it is entirely appropriate—so long as it is done opportunely, non-judgementally and never in a patronizing way—to present the emotional as well as medical advantages of delaying coitarche ('saving sex') and then of mutually faithful relationships. But even if that is medically the 'best', when rejected it must not become the enemy of the 'good', a category that surely includes contraception combined with age appropriate SRE—the latter ideally being started at home by the parent(s) and not just left to schools. Legally, following the guidance below, in the decision to prescribe a medical method of contraception, an attempt should first be made to seek parental support.

However, if the young person refuses to allow this, it can be good practice to initiate a suitable 'medical' contraceptive, ideally a LARC.

There is a useful mnemonic for the 'Fraser guidelines' regarding those under 16. They still have relevance, though issued back in 1985 shortly after the Gillick case.

Mnemonic: UnProtected SSexual InterCourse. The health care practitioner:

U Must ensure the young person **UNDERSTANDS** the potential risks and benefits of the treatment/advice given

P Is legally obliged to discuss the value of **PARENTAL** support, yet the client must know that confidentiality is respected whether or not this is given

S Should assess whether the client is likely to have **SEXUAL** intercourse without contraception

S Should assess whether the young person's physical/mental health may **SUFFER** if not given contraceptive advice or supplies

I Must consider if it is in the client's best **INTERESTS** to give contraception without parental consent

C Must respect the duty of **CONFIDENTIALITY** that should be given to a person under 16, and which is as great as that owed to any other person

If the above guidance is followed in utmost good faith, the prescription of a medical method of contraception will never be seen in law as aiding or abetting the commission of the crime of underage sex.

Some 'A's about young people and unplanned conception

A lcohol—greatest single cause (and enough on its own to justify promoting 'LARC' methods)

A ttitude & A mbience—a focus group of sexually active teens attending Brook clinics was once asked: 'Who would you like to supply your contraception?'

Their response: 'Someone with a smile would be your best bet'.

This speaks volumes about their past experiences .... Hopefully these days their provider would meet them non-judgementally, with empathy and that smile!

A buse—always a possibility to be sensitive about

A bstinence?—which is *not* a ridiculous notion

A mbition in life—isn't having this the best of all contraceptives?

SEXUALLY TRANSMITTED INFECTIONS

Taking a quick but matter-of-fact sexual history need not be stressful. It should be seen as part of the consultation for all contraceptives, not just the intrauterine ones.

In context (of discussion about sex and contraception), ask:

- 'When did you last have sex?' and then immediately
- 'When did you last have sex with anybody different?'

Much can be learnt at once from this pair of open questions, whether the response is 'about 21 years ago' ... or say '3 months ago'. If the latter, it now becomes unthreatening (unlike other approaches) to go on and clarify whether this was a change of partner or 'a one night stand'—and whether there have been others in the past year. Getting a handle on whether the woman's partner himself is monogamous or otherwise can be tricky, but if tactfully asked she may, sometimes, have a pretty good idea.

In the United Kingdom, *higher risk of infection particularly with Chlamydia trachomatis* applies to women aged under 25 and/or presenting with the request for emergency contraception. But a good history taken as above suggests even greater likelihood of a positive result if there has been:

- a partner change in the previous 12 weeks
- more than one partner in the past 12 months
- any history of having tests at a sexual health clinic.

Advise all about minimizing their risk of sexually transmitted infections (STIs), including HIV. If when counselling an individual the 'selling' of monogamy fails, *it is essential to promote the condom as an addition to their selected contraceptive, whenever (now or later) there may be an infection risk—the so-called Double-Dutch approach.*

Features of the ideal contraceptive
- 100% effective (with the default state as contraception)
- 100% convenient (can forget about it, non-coitally related)
- 100% safe, free of adverse side effects (neither risk nor nuisance)
- 100% reversible, ideally by self
- 100% maintenance-free, meaning it needs absolutely no medical or provider intervention (with potential pain or discomfort), whether initially or ongoing or to achieve reversal
- 100% protective against STIs
- Having other non-contraceptive benefits, especially to reduce the dis-'eases' of the menstrual cycle
- Cheap, easy to distribute
- Acceptable to every culture, religion and political view
- Used by or at least obviously visible to the woman, who most needs to know it has worked!

No available method meets all the criteria in the above box, though the LNG-IUS gets closest.

RELATIVE EFFECTIVENESS OF THE AVAILABLE METHODS

Failure rates of methods are usually expressed as per 100 woman-years. A figure of 10 per 100 woman-years for a 'perfect user' (see below) means that in a population of 100 users 10 women might be expected to conceive in the first year of use of the method; or, notionally, one woman would have an 'evens' chance of having an unplanned pregnancy after 10 years of its use. In Table 1, 'Perfect use' means the method is used both consistently and correctly, whereas 'Typical use' means what it says and is obviously hugely dependent on characteristics (e.g. age, social class, acceptability of conception, etc.) of the population studied. Note the huge difference in percentage conceiving after 1 year between the two types of use for the combined Pill (0.3 vs. 8). The data in this table have come from the United States, but the Perfect use data are usable for comparing methods in any setting.

Table 1

Percentage of women experiencing an unintended pregnancy during the first year of use of contraception

Method (1)	Percentage of women experiencing an unintended pregnancy within the first year of use	
	Typical use (2)	**Perfect use (3)**
No method[a]	85	85
Spermicides	29	18
Withdrawal	27	4
Fertility awareness–based methods[b]	25	
Standard days method		5
Ovulation method		3
Sponge		
Parous women	32	20
Nulliparous women	16	9
Diaphragm plus spermicide	16	6
Condom		
Female	21	5
Male	15	2
Combined Pill and progestogen-only Pill	8	0.3
Evra patch	8	0.3
NuvaRing	8	0.3
Depo-Provera	3	0.3
Combined injectable (Lunelle)	3	0.05
IUD		
ParaGard[c]	0.8	0.6
Mirena (LNG-IUS)	0.2	0.2
Implanon	0.05	0.05
Female sterilization	0.5	0.5
Male sterilization	0.15	0.10

Emergency contraceptive Pills: treatment initiated within 72 hours after unprotected intercourse reduces the risk of pregnancy by at least 75%.
Lactational amenorrhea method: LAM is a highly effective, *temporary* method of contraception.

Data from United States of America.
[a]The percentages becoming pregnant in columns (2) and (3) are based on data from populations where contraception is not used and from women who cease using contraception in order to become pregnant. Among such populations, about 89% become pregnant within 1 year. This estimate was lowered slightly (to 85%) to represent the percentage who would become pregnant within 1 year among women now relying on reversible methods of contraception if they abandoned contraception altogether.
[b]The ovulation method is based on evaluation of cervical mucus. The standard days method avoids intercourse on cycle days 8 through 19.
[c]Equivalent to the T-Safe Cu 380 A and its clones.
Source: Adapted from Trussell J. Contraceptive efficacy. In: Hatcher RA, Trussell J, Nelson AL, et al. Contraceptive Technology. 19th revised ed. New York, NY: Ardent Media, 2007.

Continuation rates also vary even among 'perfect' users and in general are much higher for the long-acting reversible methods (LARCs).

ELIGIBILITY CRITERIA FOR CONTRACEPTIVES

The World Health Organization system for classifying contraindications

This excellent scheme (first devised in a small WHO workshop that I attended in 1994, in Atlanta) is more fully described in the document issued by WHO, *Medical Eligibility Criteria for Contraceptive Use*, fourth edition (Geneva: WHO, 2009), which will be referred to from now on as WHOMEC. This is dark blue in colour and its companion volume (green) is *Selected Practice Recommendations for Contraceptive Use* (Geneva: WHO, 2004), generally referred to as WHOSPR. They are readily downloadable from www.who.int/reproductivehealth/topics/family_planning/en/index.html (click on the relevant icons for either volume). Both of these are evidence based, where evidence exists.

The FSRH's Clinical Effectiveness Unit has since developed a UK version (UKMEC) of WHOMEC, which adjusts for UK practice and so differs slightly—therefore in most (but not quite all) cases being more closely congruent with this book. UKMEC is available on the FSRH website www.fsrh.org/pdfs/UKMEC2009.pdf.

WHOMEC and UKMEC classify eligibility for contraceptive methods into four categories, as in the following box:

WHO classification of contraindications
(A–D is the author's parallel aide-memoire for the significance of each category)

1. A condition for which there is no restriction for the use of the contraceptive method
   'A' is for **Always Usable**
2. A condition where the advantages of the method generally outweigh the theoretical or proven risks
   'B' is for **Broadly Usable, Be alert** (for any future added risk)

*****

The most useful feature of the classification is the separation into two categories of 'relative' contraindication (WHO 2 and 3), with the 'strong relative' ones (WHO 3) below the line: implying that *they normally indicate non-use of the method.*

Clinical judgement is required, always in consultation with the contraceptive user, especially (1) in all WHO 3 conditions or (2) if more than one condition applies. As a working rule, two WHO 2 conditions usually move the situation to WHO 3; and if any WHO 3 condition applies, the addition of either a 2 or a 3 condition normally means WHO 4, i.e. 'Do not use'.

For all the medical methods described in the rest of this book, the listed absolute or relative contraindications are based on the above scheme. Prescribers often have to make a decision (in consultation with the woman/couple) despite a frustrating absence of good evidence.

What follows is the best interim guidance, pending more data, according to this author's judgement after assessing the evidence and the views of WHOMEC and UKMEC, if available. Note that these bodies have yet to give their verdict on some issues.

To avoid confusion, here, all categories are usually preceded herein by 'WHO' rather than 'UKMEC'—indicating use of the WHO's categorization scheme, with the chosen category being most often *but not always* identical to that currently advised in this country by UKMEC. *The few usually small differences from UKMEC and/or WHO are identified in the text by 'in my view'.*

Final introductory points:

1. The manufacturers' SPCs and PILs may also differ (from WHOMEC, from UKMEC and from what is said here . . .).
2. Use of some brand names here does *not* imply their endorsement, they are only used for ease of reference.
3. There is a Glossary in the Appendix for all abbreviations.

CHC is not *a typo* for COC (combined oral contraceptive(s)) . . .. it means combine*d hormonal* contraceptive(s), the subject of the next chapter, and includes along with oral Pills, contraceptive patches and rings (Evra™ and NuvaRing™). It is important to note that though the evidence base is far stronger about COCs, the majority of the statements about them will also apply to the other CHCs.

Valuable information along with 195 references in support of the next chapter about the CHCs is at:
www.fsrh.org/pdfs/CEUGuidanceCombinedHormonalContraception.pdf

For more specific information about the skin patch and vaginal ring CHC methods, please visit:
www.fsrh.org/pdfs/ProductReviewEVRA.pdf and: www.fsrh.org/pdfs/CEUStatementNexplanon1110.pdf

Combined hormonal contraception

COMBINED ORAL CONTRACEPTIVES
Mechanism of action

The combined oral contraceptive (COC) Pills currently available in the United Kingdom are shown in Table 2. They combine an estrogen [ethinylestradiol (EE) in all cases but one] with one of eight progestogens.

Aside from secondary contraceptive effects on the cervical mucus and to impede implantation, COCs primarily prevent ovulation. This makes the method highly effective in 'perfect' use (Table 1), but it removes the normal menstrual cycle and replaces it with a cycle that is user produced and based only on the end organ, i.e. the endometrium. So the withdrawal bleeding has minimal medical significance, can be deliberately postponed or made infrequent or abolished (e.g. tricycling and 365/365 Pill-taking, discussed below); and if it fails to occur, once pregnancy is excluded, poses no problem. The Pill-free time is the contraception-deficient time, which has great relevance to advice for the maintenance of COC efficacy (see below).

Benefits vs. risks

Capable of providing virtually 100% protection from unwanted pregnancy and taken at a time unconnected with sexual activity, the COC provides enormous reassurance by the associated regular, short, light and usually painless withdrawal bleeding at the end of the 21-day pack. Inevitably, most of this section will focus on possible risks and hazards associated with taking the

Table 2

Formulations of currently marketed combined oral contraceptives, in the UK

Pill type	Brand names available (in United Kingdom[a])	Estrogen (µg)	Progestogen (µg)	
Monophasic				
Ethinylestrogen/ Norethisterone	Loestrin 20	20	1000	Norethisterone acetate[b]
	Loestrin 30	30	1500	Norethisterone acetate[b]
	Brevinor	35	500	Norethisterone
	Ovysmen	35	500	Norethisterone
	Norimin	35	1000	Norethisterone
Ethinylestrogen/ levonorgestrel	Microgynon 30 (and ED version) Rigevidon Levest Ovranette	30	150	
Ethinylestrogen/ desogestrel	Mercilon Gedarel 20/150	20	150	
	Marvelon Gedarel 30/150	30	150	
Ethinylestrogen/ gestodene	Femodette 20/75 Sunya 20/75 Millinette 20/75	20	75	
	Femodene (and ED) Katya 30/75 Millinette 30/75	30	75	
Ethinylestrogen/ norgestimate	Cilest	35	250	
Ethinylestrogen/ drospirenone	Yasmin	30	3000	
Mestranol/ norethisterone[c]	Norinyl-1	50	1000	
Bi/triphasic				
Ethinylestrogen/ norethisterone	BiNovum	35	500 } 833[d]	(7 tabs)
		35	1000 }	(14 tabs)
	Synphase	35	500 }	(7 tabs)
		35	1000 } 714	(9 tabs)
		35	500 }	(5 tabs)
	TriNovum	35	500 }	(7 tabs)
		35	750 } 750	(7 tabs)
		35	1000 }	(7 tabs)
Ethinylestrogen/ levonorgestrel	Logynon (and ED) TriRegol	30 }	50 } 92	(6 tabs)
		40 } 32[d]	75 }	(5 tabs)
		30 }	125 }	(10 tabs)
Ethinylestrogen/ gestodene	Triadene	30 }	50 }	(6 tabs)
		40 } 32	70 } 79	(5 tabs)
		30 }	100 }	(10 tabs)
Estradiol valerate/ dienogest	Qlaira	3000		(2 tabs)
		2000	2000	(5 tabs)
		2000	3000	(17 tabs)
		1000		(2 tabs)
		Inert	Inert	(2 tabs)
Ethinylestrogen/ cyproterone acetate (co-cyprindiol[e])	Dianette Clairette Acnocin Cicafem	35	2000	

[a]Other names in use worldwide are on the website www.ippf.org.
[b]Converted to norethisterone as the active metabolite.
[c]Has to be converted to ethinylestradiol, approximately 35 µg, as active estrogen, so Norinyl-1 approximates to Norimin (see text).
[d]Equivalent daily doses per formulation in these columns, for comparison with monophasic brands.
[e]Marketed primarily as acne therapy, not as a standard COC.

Pill, but the positive aspects should not be forgotten; they are listed in the box below. Although some of these findings await full confirmation, the good news is rarely mentioned while the suspected risks are widely publicized and often over-dramatized.

Space does not allow full discussion of all the work that has been published in the half-century during which the Pill has been available in this country. Practitioners should form their own opinion of the risks and benefits by their own reading, but the following may help to summarize present medical opinion upon which contemporary prescription of the Pill is based.

The data presented here have been derived from the prospective Royal College of General Practitioners (RCGP), Oxford/fpa and US Nurses Studies, supplemented by numerous case-control studies and a few randomized controlled trials conducted by the WHO and other bodies.

Contraceptive benefits of COCs
- Effectiveness
- Convenience, not intercourse related
- Reversibility

Non-contraceptive benefits of COCs
These at times may provide the principal indication for use of the method (e.g. in the treatment of severe primary dysmenorrhoea in a not-yet sexually active teenager).
- Reduction of *most menstrual cycle disorders*: less heavy bleeding, therefore less anaemia, and less dysmenorrhoea; regular bleeding, the timing of which can be controlled (no Pill-taker ever needs to have Pill 'periods' at weekends); fewer symptoms of premenstrual tension overall; no ovulation pain
- Reduced risk of *cancer of the ovary, cancer of the endometrium* and also according to latest data, *colorectal cancer*
- Fewer *functional ovarian cysts*, because associated abnormal ovulation is prevented
- Fewer *extrauterine pregnancies*, because normal ovulation is inhibited
- Reduction in *pelvic inflammatory disease* (PID)
- Reduction in *benign breast disease*
- Fewer *symptomatic fibroids*
- Probable *reduction in thyroid disease*, whether over- or under-activity

- Probable reduction in risk of *rheumatoid arthritis*
- Fewer *sebaceous disorders*, especially acne (with estrogen-dominant COCs such as Marvelon™ and Yasmin™)
- Possible reduced risk of *endometriosis* (a potential benefit probably not as well realized as it would be if the Pill were more commonly taken in a bleed-free regimen)
- Continuous use certainly beneficial in long-term *suppression of established endometriosis*
- Possibly *fewer duodenal ulcers* (not well established)
- Reduction in *Trichomonas vaginalis* infections
- Possible lower incidence of *toxic shock syndrome*
- *No toxicity* in overdose
- Some *obvious beneficial social effects*, to balance the suggested negatives

Even as we turn to unwanted effects, it is reassuring that, based, inter alia, on the regular reports of the RCGP study ever since it began in 1968, COCs have their main (small) effect on every known associated cause of mortality during current use and for some (variable) time thereafter. The excess thrombotic risk has probably vanished by 4 weeks, and by 10 years after use ceases, all-cause mortality in past-users is lower than or (allowing for healthy-user bias) certainly indistinguishable from that in never-users.

Tumour risk and COCs

No medication continues to receive so much scrutiny and investigation as the Pill. Fears have been expressed for many years about its possible connection with breast, cervical and (rare) primary liver cancers.

Breast cancer

The incidence of this disease is high, and therefore it must inevitably be expected to develop in women whether they take COCs or not. Since the recognized risk factors include early menarche and late age of first birth, use by young women was rightly bound to receive scientific scrutiny. The literature to date has been copious, complex, confusing and often contradictory!

The 1996 publication by the Collaborative Group on Hormonal Factors in Breast Cancer reanalysed original data relating to over

53,000 women with breast cancer and over 100,000 controls from 54 studies in 25 countries. This is 90% of the world epidemiological data. The reanalysis showed disappearance of the risk in ex-users, but *recency of use* of the COC was shown to be the most important factor: with the odds ratio unaffected by age of initiation or discontinuation, use before or after first full-term pregnancy, duration of use, or dose. The main findings are summarized in Table 3. Figure 2 shows that the background risk of cancer under the age of 35 is, fortunately, very small. Hence, for the age group who most often use the method, the absolute numbers affected even for current users with the highest added risk in Table 3 is actually small.

A 2002 study of 4575 breast cancer patients and matched cancer-free controls in the United States was congruent with this and

Table 3

The increased risk of developing breast cancer while taking the Pill and in the 10 years after stopping

User status	Percentage increased risk
Current user	24%
1–4 years after stopping	16%
5–9 years after stopping	7%
10 plus years an ex-user	No significant excess risk

Source: From Collaborative Group on Hormonal Factors in Breast Cancer. Lancet 1996; 347:1713–1727.

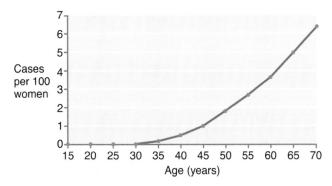

Figure 2
Background risk: cumulative number of breast cancers per 100 women, by age.
Source: From statement by the Faculty of Family Planning—now FSRH—June 1996.

particularly reassuring in that there was nothing to suggest the so-called time-bomb problem: namely, despite 75% exposure to the COC in the population, there was *no persistence of risk in long-time ex-users* when they reached ages with much higher incidence of this cancer, as shown in Figure 2. This finding remains valid to date (2012), after taking account of all subsequent reports.

COC-users can be reassured that
- While the small increase in breast cancer risk for women on the Pill noted in previous studies is confirmed, the odds ratio of 1.24 signifies an increase of 24% only while women are taking the COC, diminishing to zero after discontinuation, over the next few years.
- Beyond 10 years after stopping, there is no detectable increase in breast cancer risk for former Pill-users.
- The cancers diagnosed in women who use or have ever used COCs are clinically less advanced than those who have never used the Pill, and are less likely to have spread beyond the breast.
- These risks are not associated with duration of use, or the dose or type of hormone in the COC, and there is no synergism with other risk factors for breast cancer (e.g. family history).
- If 1000 women use the Pill till age 35, by age 45 this model (which itself is a 'worst-case scenario') shows there will be, in all, 11 cases of breast cancer. Importantly, though, as displayed in Figure 3, only one of these cases is extra (i.e. Pill related), the others would have arisen anyway, in a control group of 1000 never-users.

Clinical implications   The breast cancer issue should be addressed, in a sensitive way, as part of routine Pill counselling for all women.

This discussion should be initiated opportunely—not necessarily at the first visit if not raised by the woman—along with encouragement to report promptly any unusual changes in their breasts at any time in the future ('breast awareness'). The balancing protective effects against other malignancies (see below) should also be mentioned.

The known contraceptive and non-contraceptive benefits of COCs may seem so great to many (but not to all) as to compensate for almost any likely lifetime excess risk of breast cancer.

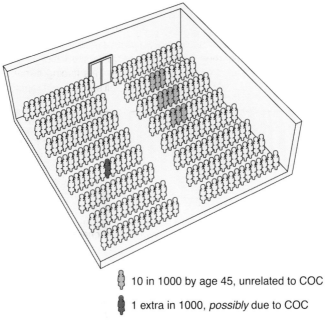

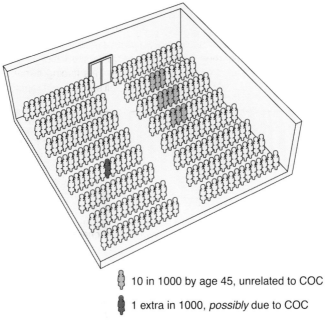 10 in 1000 by age 45, unrelated to COC

 1 extra in 1000, *possibly* due to COC

Figure 3
Cumulative incidence of breast cancer during and after use of COC until age 35.

- *What about Pill use by older women?* There is no change in relative risk, but an increased attributable risk (3 extra cases per 1000 for 10th year ex-users stopping at 45 and now aged 55, instead of the above 1 extra case per 1000 for 10th year ex-users now 45). This needs explaining and may be acceptable to many, given the balancing (see below) from the well-established protection against cancers of the ovary, endometrium, colon and rectum—and their incidence also increases with age. However, the majority of women would now probably prefer one of the newer options available (such as the IUS or banded copper IUD, see below).
- *Women with benign breast disease (BBD) or with a family history of a young first-degree relative with breast cancer under age 40* have a larger background risk than the generality of women—but only the same as women slightly older than their current age who are free of the risk factor. This equates to a small shift of the curve to the left in Figure 2. UKMEC classifies both of these conditions as WHO 1 for the COC (no restriction on use).

- If the woman with BBD had a breast biopsy, the histology should be obtained: if the *rare pre-malignant epithelial atypia* was found, the COC should not be used (WHO 4).
- *Carriers of known gene mutations (e.g. BRCA1)* associated with this cancer should also normally avoid the COC (WHO 3).
- *If a woman develops carcinoma of the breast*, COCs should be discontinued, and women with a personal history of this cancer should avoid COCs (WHO 4). UKMEC allows COC use after 5 years of remission.

Cervical cancer

Human papillomavirus (HPV), especially types 16 and 18, appears to be the principal carcinogen for this cancer, which is clearly transmitted sexually. Systematic reviews of the studies lead to the conclusion that the COC acts as a cofactor, possibly speeding transition through the stages of cervical intraepithelial neoplasia (CIN). The raised odds ratio is further increased with increasing durations of use. As a cofactor, the COC acts similarly to, but is certainly weaker than, cigarette smoking.

Clinical implications
- Prescribers must ensure that COC-users and ex-users are adequately screened following agreed guidelines. Even if they also smoke, a 3-yearly smear frequency starting from age 25, as in national guidelines, is still believed to suffice to identify—and then treat appropriately—the vast majority (though no screening programme can have 100% success) in the pre-invasive stages, before actual cancer develops.
- It is acceptable practice (WHO 2) to continue COC use during the careful monitoring of any abnormality, or after definitive treatment of CIN.

The relative importance of any adverse effect of the COC on cervical cancer should be further minimized in future by widespread HPV vaccination to reduce the incidence, also HPV triage for borderline and mild dyskaryosis to improve pre-cancer detection.

Liver tumours

COC use increases the relative risk of *benign adenoma or hamartoma*, either of which can cause pain or rarely a haemoperitoneum. Most reported cases have been in long-term users of relatively high-dose Pills that are now not used. Moreover, the background incidence is so small (1–3 per 1 million women per year) that the COC-attributable risk is minimal.

Case-control studies support the view that the rare *primary hepatocellular carcinoma* is also minimally less rare in COC-users than in controls. Yet there is reassuring contrary evidence to the association being causative, namely that, although this cancer is usually rapidly fatal, the death rate from it has not changed detectably in either the United States or Sweden, where the COC has been widely used since the 1960s. Moreover, there is no evidence of synergism with either cirrhosis or hepatitis B liver infection.

Clinical implications
A past history of tumour (benign or malignant) is WHO 4 for the COC but WHO 3 for other forms of hormonal contraception.

Choriocarcinoma or other forms of gestational trophoblastic disease—no problem

In the presence of active trophoblastic disease, early studies from the United Kingdom showed that chemotherapy for choriocarcinoma was more often required among women given COCs. But studies in the United States have since reported the very opposite (more rapid decrease of β-hCG levels post-partum in COC-users). After consideration of all available evidence, WHO and UKMEC now both say this is WHO 1, for any hormonal method. But avoid use of any intrauterine methods (WHO 4) if there is frank malignancy or persistently elevated β-hCG levels, as there may be an increased risk of perforation.

Carcinomas of the ovary and of the endometrium

The good news is that both are definitely less frequent in COC-users. Numerous studies have shown that the incidence of both is roughly halved among all users, and reduced to one-third in long-term users; a protective effect can be detected in ex-users for up to 10 to 15 years. Suppression of ovulation in COC-users and of normal mitotic activity in the endometrium are the accepted explanations of these findings.

> **Clinical implications** It would be reasonable for a woman known to be predisposed to either of these cancers to choose to use the COC primarily for this protective effect.

Colorectal cancer

More than one study now suggests a significantly reduced risk for this cancer. In the RCGP study, the relative risk for current COC-users plus those whose last use was less than 5 years earlier was 0.49, with greater protection in long-term users. However, so far the studies have not been able to show a long-term protective effect among ex-users.

Other cancers

Associations have been mooted but not confirmed.

> **Moreover, clinically:**
> Women who are apparently cured by local radical surgery for neoplasia of the ovary, cervix and uterus and for malignant melanoma may all use COCs (WHO 2).

Benefits and risks—a summary

To summarize, in the words of the RCGP study (2009), oral contraception *'was not associated with a significantly increased risk of any cancer ... These results suggest that, at least in this relatively healthy UK cohort, the cancer benefits associated with oral contraception outweigh the risks'*. See Figure 4.

Circulatory disease and choice of COC

Venous thromboembolism

A massive UK 'Pill-scare' in 1995 could have been minimized if the data had been presented as a *reduction* in risk of venous thromboembolism (VTE) for women using levonorgestrel (LNG) or norethisterone (NET) Pills, in comparison with COCs containing the 'third-generation' progestogens desogestrel (DSG) and gestodene (GSD). This would have been presentationally better. But it would also have been scientifically more valid, as that is where the difference lies (Fig. 5): the *different* progestogens are really LNG and to a lesser extent NET.

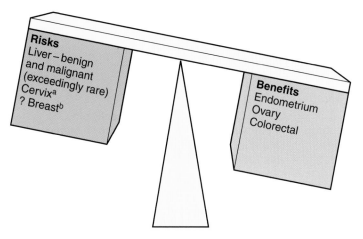

[a]COC is a weak co-factor to HPV as the *oncogen*. Cancer risk minimised *further by good practice (HPV vaccination, screening)*

[b]Possible small excess risk linked to current or recent COC-use, but no excess mortality shown in ex-takers. See text.

Figure 4
Cancer and COCs: a balance.

LNG has been shown (Fig. 5) to oppose any estrogen-mediated rise in sex hormone–binding globulin (SHBG) and in high-density lipoprotein (HDL) cholesterol—and can even lower the latter if enough is given. Somatically, it also opposes the tendency for estrogen to improve acne. It is thus unlike most other marketed progestogens, which basically allow estrogen to 'do its own thing' in a dose-dependent way. Researchers in the Netherlands and the United Kingdom have now shown that LNG when combined with EE reduces the procoagulant effects of the latter on acquired activated protein C resistance and the reduction of protein S levels. Hence, it is no longer biologically implausible that the combination of LNG with EE might (slightly) reduce the clinical risk of venous thrombosis to below what it would be with a given dose of EE alone. It looks as though DSG and GSD, and indeed most of the other progestogens used for contraception, *simply fail to have that opposing action—just as they do when we actually want a greater estrogenic effect:* when choosing a Pill for someone with acne, for example, where higher rather than lower SHBG levels help through binding circulating androgens.

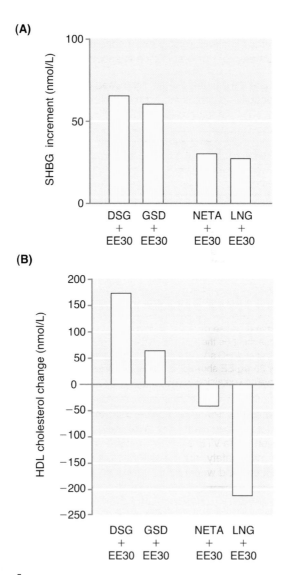

Figure 5
*Prospective randomized controlled trials of four Pills: desogestrel (DSG) + ethinyl-estradiol (EE) 30; gestodene (GSD) + EE30; norethisterone acetate (NETA) + EE30; levonorgestrel (LNG) + EE30. (**A**) Increment in sex hormone–binding globulin (SHBG). (**B**) Change in high-density lipoprotein (HDL) cholesterol. Guillebaud J. Margaret Pyke Centre Study, 2000.*

Figure 5A thus confirms clinical experience over many years that LNG COCs are not the best choice in sebaceous disorders.

Norgestimate (NGM), the progestogen used in Cilest and Evra[TM], the contraceptive patch, is in part metabolized to LNG. Yet both these two combination products with EE seem to be clinically more estrogen dominant than Microgynon 30[TM].

Any beneficial effect of LNG (and NET and its pro-drugs) on VTE risk is most probably less than the epidemiology in 1995–1996 suggested. This is because of the influence of prescriber bias, the 'healthy-user' effect and so-called 'attrition of the susceptibles'—which led, at the time of the studies, to
- women at lower intrinsic risk being more likely to be left using the older LNG or NET Pills—because the women with risk factors such as smoking and high body mass index (BMI) had been switched to what were thought to be the 'safer' newer products with which they were compared! Hence (the mirror image):
- women at higher intrinsic risk tending through prescriber bias to be using DSG and GSD products, and also for new users (always an unknown quantity with respect to predisposition to VTE) to be started on these or restarted after a break from the method. These must be the non-causative explanations for the bizarre finding in WHO's VTE study of 1995 that Mercilon[TM] containing only 20 μg EE showed an apparently greater risk of VTE than Marvelon containing 30 μg.

Clinical implications The advice from the UK Department of Health (DoH), issued after the 1998 review by the Medicines Commission of the VTE issue, started with the comment that they 'found no new safety concerns' about third-generation DSG or GSD products, and went on:

The spontaneous incidence of VTE in healthy non-pregnant women (not taking any oral contraceptive) is about 5 cases per 100,000 women per year. The incidence in users of second-generation Pills is about 15, (revised in 2011 to 20) per 100,000 women per year of use. The incidence in users of third-generation Pills is about 25 (revised to 40 in the 2011 advice) cases per 100,000 women per year of use: this excess incidence has not been satisfactorily explained by bias or confounding. The level of all of these risks of VTE increases with age and is likely to be increased in women with other known risk factors for VTE, such as obesity.

> *'Women must be fully informed of these very small risks... Provided they are, the type of Pill is for the woman together with her doctor or other family planning professionals jointly to decide in the light of her individual medical history.'* (Author's emphasis.)
> DoH 7 April 1999

The European Medicines Agency stated in June 2011 *'the risk of venous thromboembolism (VTE) for drospirenone-containing combined oral contraceptives (COCs), including Yasmin, is higher than for levonorgestrel-containing COCs (so-called "second generation" Pills) and may be similar to the risk for COCs that contain desogestrel or gestodene (so-called "third generation" Pills)'*

(See: www.ema.europa.eu/docs/en_GB/document_library/Report/2011/05/WC500106708.pdf)

They went on to confirm the above 1999 statement about *idiopathic* VTE, using updated incidence numbers for DSG, GSD [and now drospirenone (DSP)] and wording their advice for health care professionals almost identically.

The above absolute rates of VTE are still much disputed by some authorities, and by the manufacturers of DSG, GSD and DSP products. Even if, despite the issues of prescriber bias, etc., the whole difference is accepted as real, Table 4 and Figure 6, where the denominator is per million rather than per 100,000, help to put the risks into perspective:

- Using the incidence rates given above, each year there will be 200 fewer cases of VTE per million users of an LNG product such as Microgynon 30 than among a similar number of women using any 'LNG-lacking', hence more estrogen-dominant, product. Using an estimate of 1% for VTE mortality in the United Kingdom (revised downwards, see footnotes to Table 4), this means a 2 per million greater annual VTE mortality for such a product than say Microgynon 30. From Figure 6, this risk difference is the same as that from 2 hours of driving.
- Hence, if a woman chooses (as she might very reasonably do, after counselling) to control a symptom such as acne by switching away from Microgynon 30 to a product using DSG, GSD or DSP, all she needs to do is avoid a 2-hour drive in the whole of the next year to remain, in terms of VTE risk, effectively still on the Microgynon 30!

Table 4
Comparative risks

Estimated annual risks per 1,000,000 women		
Activity	**Cases**	**Deaths**
Having a baby, UK (all direct causes of death)		50
Having a baby (VTE)[a]	600	10
Using DSG/GSD/DSP Pill (VTE)[a]	400	4
Using LNG/NET Pill (VTE)[a]	200	2
Non-user, non-pregnant (VTE)[a]	50–100	<1
Risk from all causes through COC (healthy non-smoking woman), *current*[b] COC-takers		5
Home accidents		30
Playing soccer		40
Road accidents		80
Parachuting (10 jumps/year)		200
Scuba diving		220
Hang-gliding		1500
Cigarette smoking (in next year if aged 35)		1670
Death from pregnancy/childbirth in rural Africa		$\geq$ 10,000

[a]VTE rates are for idiopathic cases, with no other risk factor. VTE mortality rate assumed to be 2% in last edition, latest UK figures <1% though higher in pregnancy: hence new estimates in right hand column.

[b]Emphasis on *current* takers and more recent data (2010). The excess mortality is acceptably small in context with the other activities shown, but is moreover so much balanced in a reproductive lifetime by the mortality benefits (e.g. in cancer, see text) as to make *all-cause mortality in past-users the same or possibly even less than for never-users* (see p. 22).

Sources: Dinman BD. JAMA 1980; 244:1226–1228; Mills A, et al. BMJ 1996; 312:121; Anon. BMJ 1991; 302:743; Strom B. Pharmacoepidemiology. 2nd ed. Chichester: Wiley, 1994:57–65; www.patient.co.uk/doctor/Maternal-Mortality.htm; www.ema.europa.eu/docs/en_GB/document_library/Report/2011/05/WC500106708.pdf

- The risk difference is tiny but some of it at least is probably real—and therefore worth minimizing (why take any avoidable extra risk?) by the current UK policy of generally commencing with a LNG product as first line, while being fully prepared to switch for symptom control upon request.

- In sum, the primary reason for choosing, or changing to, a more estrogenic product, such as one containing DSG or GSD as the progestogen, is for the control of side effects occurring on a LNG or NET product.

Arterial diseases: acute myocardial infarction, haemorrhagic stroke and ischaemic stroke

Epidemiology, spearheaded by the WHO, has shown that the COC was not the prime cause of most of the arterial events occurring in Pill-takers, both within and outside research studies.

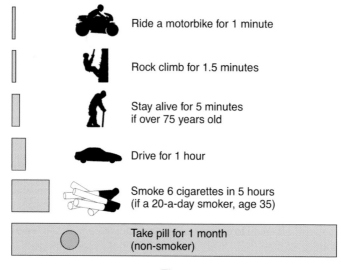

Ride a motorbike for 1 minute

Rock climb for 1.5 minutes

Stay alive for 5 minutes
if over 75 years old

Drive for 1 hour

Smoke 6 cigarettes in 5 hours
(if a 20-a-day smoker, age 35)

Take pill for 1 month
(non-smoker)

Time

Figure 6

Time required to have a 1:1,000,000 risk of dying. Source: Adapted and updated in 2010 from Minerva, British Medical Journal, 1988.

The COC was blamed, yet arterial disease is exceptionally rare in COC-takers during the reproductive years, aside from an increasing risk with age, unless they also smoke or have diabetes or hypertension. *Migraine with aura* is a specific, independent risk factor for ischaemic stroke.

- **Acute myocardial infarction (AMI)**. The relative risk or odds ratio (OR) of this condition in some studies goes up from unity (no added risk) in non-smoking controls to 10 or more in smokers also taking the COC: who indeed are in double jeopardy, since the case-fatality rate of AMI when it occurs in smokers who use the COC is also much higher.
- **Haemorrhagic stroke (HS), including subarachnoid haemorrhage**. The WHO and other studies have failed to show any increased risk due to the COC under age 35 unless there is also a risk factor such as hypertension (OR 10) or smoking (OR 3). The risk increases with age, and this effect is magnified by current COC use, but with no effect of past use or long-duration use.

- **Ischaemic stroke (IS).** Here, even in non-smokers, there is a detectable increase in the OR due to Pill-taking in the range of 1.5 to a maximum of 2. Much of this risk seems to be focused within the subpopulation who suffer from *migraine with aura* (see below). The OR is 3 for hypertension and also 3 for smoking risk.
- **Effects of dose/type of estrogen or progestogen?** These remain uncertain and would anyway only be of clinical significance when risk factors are present, given the crucial relevance of the latter to arterial disease.

Prescribing guidelines

Current scientific evidence suggests only two prerequisites for the safe provision of COCs: a careful personal and family history with particular attention to cardiovascular risk factors, and a well-taken blood pressure (BP) (Hannaford P, Webb A. Evidence-guided prescribing of combined oral contraceptives: consensus statement. Contraception 1996; 54:125–129). To this should be added, crucially, measurement of the woman's BMI at presentation.

- Prescribers should always take a comprehensive personal and family history to exclude **absolute (WHO 4) and relative contraindications (WHO 3 and 2)** to the use of COCs (see pp. 36–38).
- A personal history of definite VTE remains an absolute contraindication to any hormonal method containing EE (including Evra or NuvaRing™), combined with any progestogen.
- The risk factors for risk of future VTE and arterial wall disease must be assessed (**see Tables 5 and 6**).
- Note that it now appears, though uncertainty persists in the literature, that smoking is an independent risk factor for VTE, , as well as arterial disease.
- Alone, one risk factor from either Table 5 or 6 is a relative contraindication (WHO 2 or 3 columns), unless it is particularly severe (WHO 4 column).
- Synergism means that if WHO 3 already applies, any additional risk factor moves the category to WHO 4 ('Do not use').
- Generally, however, COC use is acceptable on a WHO 3 basis when two WHO 2 factors apply.

The remarks and footnotes in Tables 5 and 6 are fundamental to Pill prescribing.

Table 5

Risk factors for venous thromboembolism

Risk factor	Absolute contraindication WHO 4	Relative contraindication WHO 3	Relative contraindication WHO 2	Remarks
Personal or family history (FH) of thrombophilias, *or of* venous thrombosis in sibling or parent	Past VTE event; or identified clotting abnormality in this person, whether hereditary or acquired	FH of thrombosis in parent or sibling <45 with recognized precipitating factor (e.g. major surgery, post-partum) and thrombophilia screen not available	FH of thrombotic event in parent or sibling <45 with or without a recognized precipitating factor and *normal* thrombophilia screen FH in parent or sibling ≥45 or FH in second-degree relative (classified WHO 2 but tests not indicated)	*Idiopathic* VTE in a parent or sibling <45 is an indication for a thrombophilia screen if available. The decision to undertake screening in other situations (including where there was a recognized precipitating factor) will be unusual because it is very cost-ineffective—might be done on clinical grounds, in discussion with the woman Even a normal thrombophilia screen cannot be entirely reassuring, as some predispositions are unknown
Overweight—high body mass index (BMI)	BMI ≥ 40	BMI 30–39	BMI 25–29	Totality of data re BMI support these categories in my view, contrast UKMEC 2009. See footnotes.

Immobility	Bed-bound, with or without major surgery; or leg fractured and immobilized	Wheelchair life, debilitating illness	Reduced mobility for other reason	Minor surgery such as laparoscopic sterilization is WHO 1
Varicose veins (VVs)	Imminent VV surgery or any other VV treatment with known xs risk of VTE		History of superficial vein thrombosis (SVT) in the lower limbs, no deep vein thrombosis	Pulmonary embolism does not follow SVT, although past history of SVT means some caution (WHO 2) in case it might be a marker of future VTE risk. The association with VVs per se is probably coincidental
Cigarette smoking			WHO 2 for VTE risk	On balance, the literature now suggests a VTE risk from smoking, though less than the arterial disease risk it causes
Age			>35, if relates to VTE risk alone	

Notes: 1. A single risk factor in the relative contraindication columns means preference for an LNG/NET Pill, if any COC used (as in the BNF).
2. Beware of synergism: more than one factor in either of relative contraindication columns. As a working rule, two WHO 2 conditions make WHO 3; and if WHO 3 applies (e.g. BMI 30–39), addition of either a WHO 3 or WHO 2 (e.g. reduced mobility) condition normally means WHO 4 (do not use).
3. Acquired (non-hereditary) predispositions include positive results for antiphospholipid antibodies—definitely WHO 4 since they also increase the risk of arterial events (Table 6).
4. Important *acute* VTE risk factors need to be considered in individual cases: notably, major and all leg surgery, long-haul flights and dehydration through any cause.
5. There are minor differences in the above table from UKMEC, notably my more cautious categorization of BMIs above 25, with clarity that a woman whose BMI is above 40 should avoid CHCs (WHO 4).

Table 6
Risk factors for arterial disease

Risk factor	Absolute contraindication WHO 4	Relative contraindication WHO 3	Relative contraindication WHO 2	Remarks
Family history (FH) of atherogenic lipid disorder *or* of arterial CVS event in sibling or parent	Identified familial hypercholesterolaemia in this person, persisting despite treatment	FH either of known familial lipid disorder or *idiopathic* arterial event in parent or sibling <45, and client's lipid screening result not available	Client with previous evidence of hyperlipidaemia but responding well to treatment FH of arterial event with risk factor (e.g. smoking), in parent or sibling <45, and lipid screen not available	FH of premature (<45) arterial CVS disease without other risk factors, or a known atherogenic lipid disorder in a parent or sibling, indicate fasting lipid screen, where available (then check with laboratory re clinical implication of abnormal results). Despite any FH, normal lipid screen in client *is* reassuring, means WHO 1 (unlike thrombophilia screens)
Cigarette smoking		>15 Cigarettes /day	<15 Cigarettes/day	Cut-offs here are obviously arbitrary
Diabetes mellitus (DM)	Severe, longstanding or DM complications (e.g. retinopathy, renal damage, arterial disease)	Not severe/ labile and no complications, young patient		DM is always at least WHO 3 for CHCs in my view (safer options available)

Condition				
Hypertension (consistently elevated BP, with properly taken measurements)	Systolic BP >160 mmHg Diastolic BP ≥95 mmHg	Systolic BP 140–159 mmHg Diastolic BP 90–94 mmHg if essential hypertension, well controlled	BP regularly at upper limit of normal (i.e. near to 140/90) Past history of preeclampsia (WHO 3 if also a smoker)	BP levels for categories are consistent with UKMEC but different from WHOMEC (see text)
Overweight, high body mass index (BMI)	BMI ≥ 40	BMI 30–39	BMI 25–29	High BMI increases arterial as well as venous thromboembolic risk
Migraine	Migraine with aura Migraine without aura if exceptionally severe lasting more than 72 hours despite optimal medication (see text)	Migraine without aura, IF also significant added arterial risk factors	Migraine without aura	Relates to *thrombotic stroke* risk. See text for more detail (pp. 42–43)
Age > 35	Age > 35 if a continuing smoker	Age 35–51 if ex-smoker	Age 35–51 if free of all risk factors (only WHO 2, yet even safer options are available)	In all persistent smokers, age >35 best classified as WHO 4. In ex-smokers, WHO 3 is because arterial wall damage may persist

Notes: 1. Beware of synergism: more than one factor in either of relative contraindication columns. As a working rule, two WHO 2 conditions make WHO 3; and if WHO 3 applies (e.g. smoking ≥15/day) addition of either a WHO 3 or WHO 2 (e.g. age >35) condition normally means WHO 4 (as in table).

2. In continuing smokers, COC is generally stopped at age 35, in the United Kingdom. But, given the rapid risk reduction shown in studies of complete smoking cessation, according to UKMEC ex-smokers are classified WHO 3 only until 1 year, dropping to WHO 2 thereafter. In my view, WHO 3 is the best category for ex-smokers, regardless of time since cessation at age 35.

3. WHO numbers also relate to use for contraception: use of COCs for medical indications such as PCOS often entails a different risk/benefit analysis, i.e. the extra therapeutic benefits might outweigh expected extra risks, as from a high BMI or older age, for example.

4. There are minor differences in the above table from UKMEC, notably my more cautious categorization with respect to DM and smoking.

Hereditary predispositions to VTE (thrombophilias)

Almost the only indication for screening is a strong family history of one or more siblings or parents having had a spontaneous VTE under the age of 45. This justifies testing for the genetic predispositions, including factor V Leiden (the genetic cause of activated protein C resistance), which if identified is classified as WHO 4. Even if all the results are normal, however the COC remains WHO 2 at best (Table 5), indeed the family history alone remains categorized UKMEC 3. The woman's strong family history cannot be discounted, since by no means all the predisposing abnormalities of the complex haemostatic system have yet been characterized. This is why blanket screening by any blood test is not justifiable—the cost would be prohibitive and, in terms of what matters, which is the occurrence of actual disease events, there are just too many false negatives and positives.

Acquired predispositions to VTE (thrombophilias)

Antiphospholipid antibodies, which increase both VTE and arterial disease risk (Table 6, note 4) may appear in a number of connective tissue disorders, including systemic lupus erythematosus (SLE). If identified, they absolutely contraindicate COC use (WHO 4).

Which Pills are the current 'best buys' for women?

- **First, all marketed Pills are 'in the frame' for prescribing.** Given the tiny possible difference in VTE mortality between the two 'generations', the woman's own choice (initially or at any later stage) of a DSG or GSD or other estrogen-dominant product rather than an LNG or NET one after (well-documented) discussion must be respected. 'The informed user should be the chooser'.

- **First-time users**. Despite what has just been said, it is generally agreed that a low-dose LNG or NET product should remain the usual first choice. This is in part because first-timers will include an unknown subgroup who are VTE predisposed, VTE being a more relevant consideration than arterial disease at this age. Moreover, those Pills suit the majority and cost less. [Consider also offering the use of an everyday (ED) Pill type, which can help to reduce the chance of being a 'late restarter' after the Pill-free time—see below].

- **In the presence of a single WHO 2 or 3 risk factor for venous thrombosis.** The Summary of Product Characteristics (SPCs) for COCs state that DSG/GSD products are contraindicated.

  However, if there is a clear therapeutic indication for the COC, such as the polycystic ovarian syndrome (PCOS) with moderately severe acne, a different risk-benefit balance may apply. Extra therapeutic benefits from a more estrogenic product may be judged to outweigh (on a WHO 3 basis) any expected extra risks because, for example, the woman has a BMI of 35. Relevant choices might be Marvelon 30, Yasmin or Dianette™. These probably all share the same (estrogen-dominant) category—but in my view only *because they lack LNG*, with its apparent ability to antagonize effects of EE whether unwanted (prothrombotic) or wanted (e.g. SHBG increase).

- **Women with a single definite arterial risk factor (Table 6) (e.g. smokers or diabetics)—after a number of years VTE-free use or if the COC is used at all by healthy women above the age of 35.** As we have seen, in premenopausal women, AMI is almost exclusively a disease of smokers. But the hazard is higher when such risk factors are present (the RCGP's relative risk estimate for AMI was 20.8 for smoking Pill-takers!); it increases with age, and the case-fatality rate for AMI in Pill-takers is also higher. Some studies (but not others) suggest that DSG/GSD Pills might have relative advantages for arterial wall disease. Therefore, for such higher-risk women, or women *without* any such risk factors but older, *aged 35 through to c. 51* years (the average of the menopause), using a 20 μg DSG or GSD product or the natural estrogen-containing Qlaira™ might be proposed. Any advantages in so doing are far from established, and changing to a different method altogether would usually be a better course.

- **Finally, the primary reason for ever-changing COC brands is the control of side effects, for the woman's quality of life.** If, for any indication, she moves to using a product not containing LNG or NET, it should be documented that she accepts a possible tiny increase in the risk of VTE. This can be explained as comparable to the risk of driving for 2 hours in the next year (see p. 26).

Eligibility criteria for COCs

Absolute contraindications to COCs or other combined methods (e.g. Evra)

As already mentioned, all lists of absolute or relative contra-indications in this book are based on UKMEC, with a very few differences based on the author's judgement of the evidence. Compare with the Faculty Guidance document *First Prescription of Combined Oral Contraception*, at www.fsrh.org: several important conditions below (e.g. porphyria, hypertriglyceridaemia, pemphigoid gestationis and idiopathic intracranial hypertension) are not mentioned in relation to the COC there, or in UKMEC 2009.

All conditions in this first list are WHO 4 for the COC. However, as will be shown later, for the same conditions progestogen-only Pills (POPs), including Cerazette, and other progestogen-only methods, are in most cases classified no higher than WHO 2.

---

1. **Past or present circulatory disease**
   - Any *past proven arterial or venous thrombosis*
   - Established *ischaemic heart disease or angina or coronary arteritis* (current Kawasaki disease—past history is WHO 3 or 2, depending on completeness of recovery). Also significant *peripheral vascular disease*
   - *Multiple risk factors* for venous or arterial disease
   - *Severe* single factors can also be enough for the WHO 4 category (see Tables 5 and 6):
     - *BMI ≥ 40*,
     - *BP ≥ 160/>95* and
     - *diabetes with tissue damage*
   - *Atherogenic lipid disorders* (some not all, a complex issue, take advice from an expert)
   - Known prothrombotic states:
     - i.e. any of above *congenital or acquired thrombophilias*, including *SLE if antiphospholipid antibodies positive* (or unknown). Secondary Raynaud's phenomenon indicates testing for these
     - from at least 2 (preferably 4) weeks before until 2 weeks after mobilization following *elective major surgery* (do not demand that the COC be stopped for minor surgery such as brief laparoscopy with minimal post-operative

---

immobilization) and *almost all leg surgery* (e.g. operative arthroscopy of knee, or for varicose veins)
– during *leg immobilization (e.g. after fracture)*
- *Migraine **with aura*** (described on pp. 41–43)
- Definite *aura without a headache following*
- Past *ischaemic stroke, transient ischaemic attacks*
- Past *cerebral haemorrhage*
- *Pulmonary hypertension, any cause*
- *Structural heart disease* such as valvular heart disease or shunts/septal defects is only WHO 4 if there is an *added arterial or venous thromboembolic risk* (persisting, if there has been surgery). Always discuss this with the cardiologist—could be WHO 3, especially if the patient is always anticoagulated. Important WHO 4 examples:
    – *Atrial fibrillation or flutter* whether sustained or paroxysmal—or not current but high risk (e.g. mitral stenosis)
    – *Dilated left atrium* ($>$4 cm)
    – *Cyanotic heart disease*
    – Any *dilated cardiomyopathy*; but this is classified as only WHO 2 when in full remission after a past history of any type (including pregnancy cardiomyopathy)
- In other structural heart conditions, if there is little or no direct or indirect risk of thromboembolism (this being the crucial point to check with the cardiologist), the COC is usable (WHO 3 or 2)

2. **Liver**
- *Liver adenoma, carcinoma*
- *Active liver cell disease, whenever liver function tests are currently significantly abnormal*, including infiltrations, severe chronic hepatitis B and C, and cirrhosis (though UKMEC allows WHO 1 for the latter if it is compensated, no complications)
- Past *Pill-related cholestatic jaundice*; if this was only in pregnancy and never with the COC, this can be classified WHO 2. (Contrast UKMEC, who permit WHO 3, not WHO 4 as I advise here, if the attack was Pill-related)
- During *any acute viral hepatitis*: but COCs may be resumed once liver function tests have become normal (and a clinical test of two units of alcohol consumption is tolerated)
- Dubin–Johnson and Rotor syndromes are rare benign genetic disorders of hepatic secretion. COCs like pregnancy can cause overt jaundice (Gilbert's disease is WHO 2)

Note that several of the above (e.g. 4, 5 and 8) are not necessarily permanent contraindications. Moreover, many women over the years have been unnecessarily deprived of COCs for reasons now believed to have no link, such as thrush or otosclerosis; or that would have positively benefited from the method, such as secondary amenorrhoea with hypo-estrogenism.

Relative contraindications to combined oral contraceptives (COCs)

Below are listed the relative contraindications to COCs, WHO 2 or 3, signifying that the COC method is usable in context with:

- the benefit-risk evaluation for that individual
- the acceptability or otherwise of alternatives

- sometimes with special advice (e.g. in migraine, to report a change of symptomatology) or monitoring
  In cases with excess risk of venous thrombosis (e.g. wheelchair life—WHO 3—see Table 5), if the Pill is used at all for contraception, it should perhaps be a LNG/NET variety.

Relative contraindications Please read box below in conjunction with Tables 5 and 6, which deal with the commonest issues (e.g. smoking, obesity and hypertension).

Unless otherwise stated below, COCs are WHO 2:

- *Risk factors for arterial or venous disease* (see Tables 5 and 6). These are WHO 2, sometimes 3 (e.g. in my view any BMI above 30 is at least WHO 3): *provided that only one is present* and that not of such severity as to justify WHO 4.
  – *HUS* (see above): in past history may be WHO 2 if complete recovery and not Pill associated (e.g. past *Escherichia coli* O157 infection being the established cause of past attack of HUS)
  – Diabetes (minimum category being WHO 3), hypertensive disease and migraine all deserve *separate discussion* (see below)
  – *Post-partum* during the first 3 weeks (WHO 3 due to post-delivery VTE risk, but negligible fertility anyway)
- Most *chronic congenital or acquired systemic diseases* (see below) are WHO 2.
- Risk of *altitude illness* is not more probable because a climber is on COC; but if it occurs, in its most severe forms, venous or arterial thromboembolism or patchy pulmonary hypertension are known to occur, which would contraindicate the method. Hence, women climbing to above 4500 m should be informed that the COC might increase the thrombotic component of altitude illness if that were to occur (WHO 3)—and also the risk of VTE. The COC would be WHO 3, but could be only WHO 2 in many healthy trekkers who intend always to follow the maxim 'climb high but sleep low'. More details are in BMJ 2003; 326:915–919; BMJ 2011; 343:d4943 and in Faculty Guidance (URL on p 74).
- *Sex steroid–dependent cancer in prolonged remission* (WHO 3)—prolonged is defined as after 5 years by UKMEC: prime example is breast cancer.
- If a young (<40 years of age) *first-degree relative has breast cancer* or the woman herself has *benign breast disease* (WHO 2, though UKMEC says WHO 1). Being a known carrier of one of the BRCA genes is WHO 3 (p. 20).

- *Malignant melanoma* has been shown to be unrelated so is WHO 2 for the Pill.
- During the *monitoring of abnormal cervical smears* (WHO 2).
- During and after *definitive treatment for CIN* (WHO 2).
- *Oligo/amenorrhoea* (COCs may be prescribed, after investigation—may be WHO 1, use unrestricted, if the purpose is to supply estrogen in a woman needing contraception or to control the symptoms of PCOS).
- *Hyperprolactinaemia* (WHO 3, but only for patients who are on specialist drug treatment and with close supervision).
- Sickle cell trait is WHO 1, but *homozygous sickle cell disease* is WHO 2 (although DMPA is preferred for this).
- *Inflammatory bowel disease* is WHO 2, or (my view) WHO 3 if severe, because of known VTE risk in exacerbations (WHO 4, i. e. stop COC if hospitalized). Absorption of the COC might be reduced in Crohn's disease of the small bowel, but only if it is severe with evidence of malabsorption.
- *Acute porphyria* is WHO 3 in my view, since COCs can precipitate a first attack (and 1% of attacks are fatal). Other porphyrias are WHO 2, but a non-hormone method is usually preferable.
- *Gallstones:* symptomatic, medically treated (WHO 3, but WHO 2 if are an incidental finding; or after cholecystectomy).
- Very *severe depression*, if there is a history of it seemingly being exacerbated by COCs (but unwanted pregnancies can be very depressing!—and evidence supports COCs *not* causing depression).
- Diseases that require *long-term treatment with enzyme-inducing drugs* are WHO 3 [COC is usable (see below)—but alternative contraception is preferred].
- Undiagnosed genital tract bleeding (WHO 3 until diagnosed and as necessary treated).

Intercurrent diseases

It is impossible for the lists above to include every known disease that might have a bearing (i.e. WHO 4, 3 or 2) on COC prescription, and for many the data are unavailable. A working protocol is therefore:

- First, ascertain whether or not the condition might lead to **summation** with known major adverse effects of COCs, particularly thrombotic risk. If so, this usually means WHO 4, sometimes 3.
- If there are no grounds to expect summation of risk, in most serious chronic conditions the patient can be reassured that COCs are not known to have any effect—good or bad. They may

then be used (WHO 2), though with careful monitoring and alertness for the onset of new risk factors.
- The reliable protection from pregnancy that the COC can offer is often particularly important when other diseases are present, although we do now have other reliable choices that are free of EE and therefore of thrombotic risk (e.g. Cerazette™, implants, IUDs and the IUS).

Diabetes mellitus

In general, and whether type 1 or type 2, this is generally a WHO 3 condition in my view even when there is no known overt diabetic tissue damage [cf. UKMEC, which classes well-controlled diabetes mellitus (DM) as WHO 2] (see Table 6).

Clinically, given the high circulatory disease risk, in particular, the POP (often Cerazette) or an implant are definitely preferred alternatives. These can be started following coitarche in the young; with perhaps a modern copper IUD, the LNG-IUS or sterilization to follow, as appropriate.

However, for cases where there is no known arteriopathy, retinopathy, neuropathy or renal damage, nor any added arterial risk factor such as obesity or smoking (all of which mean WHO 4)— and in my cautious view if the duration of the disease has been *less than 20 years*—Qlaira or one of the three older 20 µg EE products (Table 2) are options. These COCs should be used with due caution (WHO 3) and with the plan to switch to a preferred method as soon as acceptable.

Hypertension

Hypertension is an important risk factor for both heart disease and stroke (see Table 6).

- In most women on COCs, there is a slight increase in both systolic and diastolic BP within the normotensive range: less than 1% become clinically hypertensive with modern low doses, but the rate increases with age and duration of use. Above 140/90 mmHg, this is classified as WHO 3; but if BP is repeatedly above 160/95 (either the systolic or diastolic figure), I agree with UKMEC that the method should be stopped; and even if it then normalizes, this Pill-induced hypertension means WHO 4 for the future.

- Past severe pregnancy-induced hypertension does not predispose to hypertension during COC use, but even without this it is a risk factor for myocardial infarction (WHO 2)—markedly so if the women also smokes (WHO 3).
- Essential hypertension (not COC related), when well controlled on drugs, is WHO 3: i.e. the COC is usable, but not ideal if an effective alternative acceptable.

Migraine

Like hypertension, this condition is of critical relevance both at the first prescription and during the follow-up for all users of combined hormonal contraception (CHC).

Migraines can be defined by the answers to the following questions:

During the last 3 months did you have the following with your headaches?
1. You felt nauseated or sick in your stomach?
2. You were bothered by light a lot more than when you don't have headache.
3. Your headaches limited your ability to work, study or do what you needed to do for at least 1 day.

At least two 'yes' answers out of the three means migraine is the likely diagnosis.

From Lipton et al. A self-administered screener for migraine in primary care: The ID Migraine validation study. Neurology 2003; 61:375–382.

Migraine and stroke risk

- Studies have shown an increased risk of ischaemic stroke in sufferers of migraine *with aura* and in COC-users, and if combined, there is 'summation' of risk.
- There is good evidence of exacerbation of risk by arterial risk factors, including smoking and increasing age above 35 years.
- The presence of *aura* before (or sometimes even without) the headache is the main marker of risk of ischaemic stroke (WHO 4). But it seems increasingly likely that there is no significantly increased risk through having migraine *without aura*—though for the present this is still classified as WHO 2. Given that the 1-year prevalence of any migraine in women has been shown to be as high as 18%, it is crucial to identify the important subgroup with aura (1-year prevalence about 5%).

Migraine with aura

- Taking this crucial history starts by establishing the timing: neurological symptoms of aura begin before the headache itself, and typically last around 20 to 30 minutes (maximum 60 minutes) and stop before the headache (which may be very mild). Headache may start as aura is resolving, or there may be a gap of up to 1 hour.

- Visual symptoms occur in 99% of true auras, and hence should be asked about first.
- These are typically bright and affect part of the field of vision, on the same side in both eyes (homonymous hemianopia).
- Fortification spectra are often described, typically a bright scintillating zigzag line gradually enlarging from a bright centre on one side, to form a convex C-shape surrounding the area of lost vision (which is a bright scotoma).
- Sensory symptoms are confirmatory of aura, occurring in around one-third of cases and rarely in the absence of visual aura. Typically, they come as 'pins and needles' (paraesthesia) spreading up one arm or one side of the face or the tongue; the leg is rarely affected. They are positive symptoms—not loss of function.
- Disturbance of speech may also occur, in the form of dysphasia.

Note the absence in the above list of the symptoms that occur during headache itself (photophobia or e.g. *generalised blurring or 'flashing lights'*). Moreover, aura symptoms should not be confused with premonitory symptoms, such as food cravings, excessive lethargy, extra sensitivity to light and sound, occurring a day or so before any migraine (i.e. with or without aura) and often continuing into the headache.

Clinical implications

- Ask the woman to describe a typical attack from the very beginning, including any symptoms before a headache. Listen to what she says, but at the same time watch her carefully.
- A most useful **sign** that what she describes is likely to be true aura is if she waves her hand on one or other side of her own head and draws something like a zigzag line in the air.

Migraine-related absolute contraindications (WHO 4) to starting or continuing the COC or any CHC

- *Migraine with aura* or *aura alone with no following headache*. The artificial estrogen of the COC is what needs to be avoided (or stopped, at once and forever) to minimize the additional risk of a thrombotic stroke.
- Migraine attack *without* aura that is exceptionally severe in a woman who has just started taking a CHC, and lasting more than 72 hours despite optimal medication. Could be WHO 3 in established COC-user with migraine *without* aura once evaluated.
- All migraines treated with ergot derivatives, due to their vasoconstrictor actions. (Triptans are much preferred for most women).

Note that in all of the above circumstances, any of the progestogen-only (i.e. estrogen-free) hormonal methods may be offered immediately. Similar headaches may continue, but now without the potential added risk from prothrombotic effects of EE.

Particularly useful choices are the POP (Cerazette in the young), an implant, the LNG-IUS, or a modern copper IUD (all WHO 1 in my view, although strangely WHOMEC and UKMEC both classify the first three as WHO 2).

WHO 3. The COC is usable with caution and close supervision:

- Primarily, this means migraine *without* aura (common/simple migraine) where there are also important risk factor(s) for ischaemic stroke present. A good example is heavy smoking, which itself is a significant risk factor of ischaemic stroke.

- Secondly, a clear past history of typical migraine *with* aura more than 5 years earlier or only during pregnancy, with no recurrence, may be regarded as WHO 3. COCs may be given a trial, with counselling and regular supervision, along with a specific warning that the onset of definite aura (carefully explained) means that the user should
  - stop the Pill immediately,
  - use alternative contraception, and
  - seek medical advice as soon as possible.

Migraine: relative contraindications for the COC

WHO 2. The COC is certainly 'broadly usable' in the following cases:
- Migraine *without* aura, and also without any arterial risk factor from Table 6, even if it is the woman's first ever attack occurring while taking the COC (this is a change from previous advice). Note that if these (or indeed other 'ordinary' headaches) occur only or mainly in the Pill-free interval (PFI), tricycling or continuous use of the COC may help.
- Use of a triptan drug in the absence of any other contraindicating factors.

Differential diagnoses

It may be difficult to distinguish relatively common, migraine-associated focal neurological symptoms from rare organic episodes—true transient ischaemic attacks (TIAs). TIAs are more sudden in onset than migraine aura, and although they usually last under an hour, they often include weakness or paralysis of the face, arm or leg, which is not typical in migraine. Upon suspicion, these of course mean the same in practice, i.e. WHO 4—stop the Pill immediately. If an organic episode is a possibility, hospital investigation should also follow.

The following features are not typical of migraine

- Focal epilepsy, severe acute vertigo, hemiparesis, ataxia, aphasia or unilateral tinnitus
- A severe unexplained drop attack or collapse
- Monocular blindness (black scotoma)—this could rarely be a retinal vascular event or a symptom of TIA (amaurosis fugax)

- Progressive or persistent neurological symptoms (migraine is episodic, with complete freedom from symptoms between attacks)

The 'Pill-free interval' and its implications for COC prescribing and maintenance of efficacy

As no contraceptive is being taken during the PFI, it has important efficacy implications (Fig. 7). Biochemical and ultrasound data obtained at the MPC and elsewhere demonstrate return of significant pituitary and ovarian follicular activity during the PFI in about 20% of cases—to a marked extent in some—but even in these cases, renewed Pill-taking after no more than a 7-day PFI restores ovarian quiescence. However, these data make it clear that any lengthening of the PFI beyond 7 days is likely to lead to breakthrough ovulation. Lengthening of the PFI might be caused either side of the

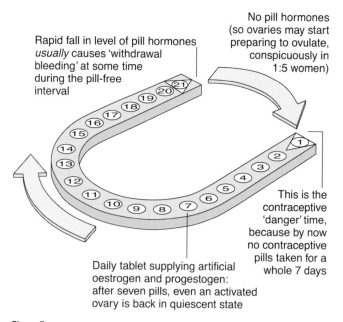

No pill hormones (so ovaries may start preparing to ovulate, conspicuously in 1:5 women)

Rapid fall in level of pill hormones *usually* causes 'withdrawal bleeding' at some time during the pill-free interval

This is the contraceptive 'danger' time, because by now no contraceptive pills taken for a whole 7 days

Daily tablet supplying artificial oestrogen and progestogen: after seven pills, even an activated ovary is back in quiescent state

Figure 7

'Horseshoe' analogy to explain the 21-day cycle. Omission of tablets either side of the gap in the horseshoe lengthens the 'contraception-losing interval' (see text).

'horseshoe' in Figure 7; i.e. from omissions, malabsorption as from vomiting (an advantage of the non-oral CHC products Evra and NuvaRing), or enzyme-inducing drug interactions that involve Pills either at the start or at the end of a packet.

All prospective COC-users need warning about this, as their initial thought is bound to be that the 'worst' Pills to miss would be in the middle of a packet (i.e. they use the wrong analogy with the middle of a normal cycle). Indeed, the 'worst Pills', actually the first two in any pack, are not seen by most COC-takers as *even being* 'missed Pills'! Starting the next pack late—given it is just after the falsely reassuring withdrawal bleed—does not trigger them even to seek advice about maintaining their contraception—unless they have been properly taught. This is why I teach that all COC Pill-takers, as they leave the surgery or clinic, should learn and repeat the *mantra*: **'I must never be a late restarter'** …. **'I must never be a late restarter'**. Moreover, let's use better the available technology, namely:

Mobile Phones. Almost all Pill-takers in the United Kingdom have one of these and most have a calendar function. Teaching about the COC, indeed all CHCs, should now include 'set your mobile to remind you every 28 days to commence a new pack (or patch, or ring)'. This is *much* more important for most women than being reminded every 24 hours to take one of the 21 active tablets. See below regarding 28-day packaging which also helps, if only by increasing the chance of the user noticing during her PFI that she needs a new supply of her method.

A population of current Pill-users was studied after the end of a routine PFI (Smith S, et al. Contraception 1986; 34:513–522). The study showed that if only 14 or even as few as 7 Pills were then taken, no fertile ovulation occurred after 7 Pills were subsequently missed. This and other work may be summarized as follows:

- Seven consecutive Pills are enough 'to shut the door' on the ovaries (therefore Pills 8–21, or longer during tricycling, simply 'keep the door shut').
- Seven Pills can be omitted without ovulation, as indeed is regularly the case in the PFI.
- More than seven Pills missed (in total) risks ovulation.

Clinical implications

The duration of clinicians' uncertainty about what advice to give women who have missed tablets is incredible: it is 50 years since the COC was first marketed in the United Kingdom! Based on another review of the evidence, the UK MHRA has at last (2011) produced what I consider acceptable advice for 'missed Pills' (see www.fsrh.org/pdfs/CEUStatementMissedPills.pdf). Moreover, the unhelpful earlier WHO, UKMEC and fpa scheme with two protocols, one for up to 20 μg EE-containing products and one for higher doses, has been abandoned.

Given the known marked individual variation in ovarian responses, which have much greater significance for efficacy than the Pill dose taken, I have always favoured instructions that err on the side of caution; so long as they are evidence based as summarized in Figure 7 and above all conveyed as simply as can be.

What follows is unchanged from what I have regularly recommended in previous editions. The definition of a 'missed Pill' is '24 hours late' (in line with WHO, though the SPCs of most manufacturers continue to say 12 hours). There are then just four bullet points to the advice that I continue to recommend:

- **'ONE tablet missed, for up to 24 hours': aside from taking the delayed Pill as soon as remembered and the next one on time, no special action is needed. This applies up to the time that two tablets would need to be taken at once.**
- **'MORE THAN ONE tablet missed' (i.e. anything more than 24 hours elapsed since an active Pill should have been taken, and a second tablet also late by one or maybe *many more* hours): *Use CONDOMS as well, for the next 7 days.***

Plus:
- **If this happened in the third active Pill week, *at the end of the pack RUN ON to the next pack* (skipping seven placebos if present).**
- **In the first Pill week, with sexual exposure since the last pack ended, EMERGENCY CONTRACEPTION (EC) is recommended IF:**
  – the user is a 'late restarter' by more than 2 days (>9-day PFI), OR
  – more than two Pills are missed in the first week, OR

> – she had a >9 day PFI through missed Pills at the end of the *last* pack.
>
> Hormonal EC should be followed, next day, by taking the appropriate day's tablet.

Figure 8 presents the same advice in a flowchart for users. In both the box and Figure 8, note my preference for the wording 'more than one Pill missed' rather than the MHRA's 'two or more Pills missed'. These are not synonymous in practice. The wording used here is both

- more cautious (as I favour: to ensure the least chance of failure with omissions of any of the crucial Pills 1–7) and
- makes it completely clear that a woman who is late with one tablet by (say) 36 hours and a second one also, but so far by only 12 hours, should begin to use condoms for any sex.

Almost all current and past advice is over-cautious for missed Pills later than the first week. In the third week, if a Pill-user omits three to four Pills and does follow the instruction to miss her next routine PFI by running on to the next pack, she will be even less likely to ovulate than usual.

In the second week, the seven or more Pills she has taken will have made her ovary quiescent after the previous PFI, so three to four tablets missed should not be enough to allow ovulation. Hence, the advice to use condoms for 7 days is highly fail-safe: if a woman worries that it was not followed, EC would only be needed if the history suggests seriously erratic Pill-taking, earlier, as well.

If 28-day packs are used (e.g. Microgynon ED, which usefully helps to avoid risky 'late restarts'), the user must learn which are the dummy 'reminder' tablets. If she misses some of the last seven (yellow) active Pills, she must be taught to omit all the (white) placebos.

After Pill-taking errors or severe vomiting or short-term use of an enzyme-inducer drug (see below), all women should be asked to report back if they have no withdrawal bleeding in the next PFI.

Every time you miss any one pill (late by up to 24 hours):

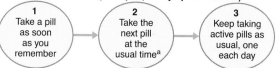

1
Take a pill as soon as you remember

2
Take the next pill at the usual time[a]

3
Keep taking active pills as usual, one each day

If you miss more than 1 pill – meaning anything *more* than 24 hours have elapsed since the time an active pill should have been taken:

4
As well as 1–3, avoid sex or use an extra method for 7 days[b] and:

In these special cases, ALSO follow these special rules:

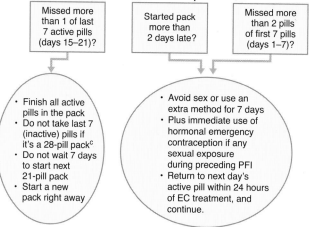

Missed more than 1 of last 7 active pills (days 15–21)?

Started pack more than 2 days late?

Missed more than 2 pills of first 7 pills (days 1–7)?

- Finish all active pills in the pack
- Do not take last 7 (inactive) pills if it's a 28-pill pack[c]
- Do not wait 7 days to start next 21-pill pack
- Start a new pack right away

- Avoid sex or use an extra method for 7 days
- Plus immediate use of hormonal emergency contraception if any sexual exposure during preceding PFI
- Return to next day's active pill within 24 hours of EC treatment, and continue.

If you miss any of the 7 inactive pills (in a 28-pill[c] pack only):

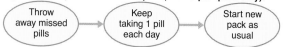

Throw away missed pills

Keep taking 1 pill each day

Start new pack as usual

[a]This can mean taking two pills at once, both at the time when you would normally take the next scheduled one. (But if it is any later, see the 'more than 1 pill' advice.)

[b]9 days for Qlaira—*plus* see text.

[c]28-pill (ED) packs can obviously help some pill-takers not to forget to restart after each PFI (the contraception-losing interval) (see text). Even with triphasic pills, you should go straight to (the first phase of) the same brand. You may bleed a bit but you will still strengthen your contraception.

Figure 8

Advice for missed Pills. (Regarding Pill days 8 to 14, see p. 49.)

Vomiting and diarrhoea

If vomiting began over 2 hours after a Pill was taken, it can be assumed to have been absorbed. Otherwise, follow the advice in the box on page 48 or Figure 8, according to the number and timing of the tablets deemed to have been missed. Diarrhoea alone is not a problem, unless it is of cholera-like severity.

Previous COC failure

Women who have had a previous COC failure may claim perfect compliance or perhaps admit to omission of no more than one Pill. Either way, as surveys show, most women miss a tablet quite frequently yet rarely conceive, so Pill failure tells us more about the individual's physiology than her memory. She is likely to be a member of that one-fifth of the population whose ovaries show above-average return to activity in the PFI. Such women may well be advised to choose a LARC, but could also use one of the extended regimens of Pill-taking (see below).

Once it has been appreciated that the Achilles' heel of the COC is the PFI, the COC can always be made 'stronger' as a contraceptive, by eliminating and/or shortening the PFI through numerous variations on the tricycling theme depicted in Figure 9.

Regimens for extended COC-taking

For many years, in the short term, the gap between packets of monophasic brands has often been omitted at the woman's choice, to avoid a 'period' on special occasions and on holidays.

This practice is approved and appears in most SPCs and PILs. Users of phasic Pills who wish to postpone withdrawal bleeds must use the final phase of a spare packet, or Pills from an equivalent formulation, e.g. Microgynon 30 immediately after the last tablet of Logynon^{TM}.

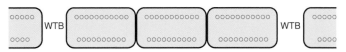

Figure 9

Tricycling (three or four—or more—packs in a row). Note the use of monophasic packs—as in Seasonale which equates to four packs in a row. Duration of PFI may also be shortened from 7 to 4 days (see text). Abbreviation: WTB, withdrawal bleeds.

Why have any PFIs at all?

The Pill-free week does promote a withdrawal bleed which some women prefer and find reassuring. Indeed, if it does not occur as expected in two successive cycles, it is standard teaching to eliminate pregnancy using a sensitive urine hCG test. However, this hormone-withdrawal bleed is irrelevant to maintaining health. So there is another group of women who are delighted not to have it—and moreover may wish to obtain the other advantages listed in the 'Extended Use' box below by simply omitting most or all the PFIs, as a long-term option (Fig. 9).

Note that no form of long-term extended use is as yet (2012) licensed in the United Kingdom. However, in the United States, Seasonale™ is a dedicated tricycle-type packaging that provides four packets of the formulation of Microgynon/Ovranette in a row, followed by a 7-day Pill-free week, such that the user has a bleed every 3 months (i.e. seasonally!). This variant requires 16 packets a year, as compared with the usual 13 packs. Seasonique is similar, with added estrogen-only during the 3-monthly PFI of 7 days. Since 30 μg EE Pills are used by these tricycling brands, the annual ingested dose is obviously greater than in traditional 21/28 regimens. So they cannot be expected to *reduce* the risks of major or minor side effects—though the prospective user may be advised that there is no evidence that it will significantly increase them, either.

Since 2003, mainly in America (North and South) there have been a number of promising randomized controlled studies (RCTs) of lower doses (usually 20 μg EE) comparing absolutely continuous (365/365) Pill-taking with the traditional method. These have demonstrated acceptable bleeding patterns for most (not all) users—including, in Leslie Miller's study Obstet Gynec 2003; 101:653–661, no bleeding at all in 72% of continuing users at 9 to 10 months (though there was a high drop-out rate). Unlike tricycling, using 20 μg Pills these regimens entail taking *less EE* in a year than any 30 μg COC taken the traditional 21/28 way (see box).

Continuous low-dose Pills seem to work best, and based on Miller's work continuous EE 20 μg/LNG 90 μg has arrived on some markets as Lybrel™ (or Anya™) since 2008. Edelman et al. Obstet Gynecol 2006; 107:657–665 in an RCT of LNG versus NET formulations found that sustained use of a Pill equivalent to the Loestrin 20™ in the United Kingdom was better than the EE 20 μg with LNG product for producing amenorrhoea. Therefore, pending marketing of a dedicated product in the United Kingdom—something many prescribers and users would welcome—selected women who wish to do so may try taking Loestrin 20 continuously—*on an unlicensed basis* (pp. 173–175). Though not yet formally tested, other 20 (or 30) μg EE COCs might also be used, similarly, always with warning that light, usually, but unpredictable spotting occurs—especially early on.

Some potential advantages of extended (365/365) COC regimens—e.g. using Loestrin 20

- More convenient + option maybe, once no bleeding, of more sex!
- Cheaper, less sanitary protection needed (if oligo-amenorrhoea achieved)
- Good wherever there is suspicion of decreased efficacy
- Much greater margin for errors in Pill-taking
- Less confusing 'rules': indeed, missed-Pill advice (up to 7 tablets) boils down to one instruction, simply 'return to regular Pill-taking'!
- Useful option in long-term enzyme-inducer therapy (discussed below)
- *Lower* annual dose of EE if 20 μg for all 365 days (7300 μg), than 30 μg taken 21/28 (8190 μg)
- Maintained or likely improved *non-contraceptive benefits.*

Already shown:
- Fewer cyclical symptoms [especially *fewer headaches* in the PFI and *less COC-related premenstrual syndrome* (PMS) reported]
  - *No heavy or painful COC-withdrawal bleeds*
  - *Less anaemia*

Needing confirmation epidemiologically:
  - Cancer prevention (see pp. 22–23)
  - Endometriosis—expected to be particularly good for this (both as to prevention and for maintenance therapy)
  - In epilepsy, sustained hormone levels may reduce seizure frequency.

With slight modification, most of these advantages are *also* to be expected, if the woman prefers to bleed periodically by tricycling.

Unacceptable bleeding with extended COC use

For the user of either 365/365 or any tricycling regimen, there is a method of dealing with undesired bleeding which is usually effective. She is advised, in advance, that if the duration of any such bleeding is unacceptable, e.g. more than 4 days, she can at any time (so long as >7 Pills have been taken consecutively) simply let the bleeding trigger her to take a break from Pill-taking—for 3 (or 4) days. This is empowering (*Sisters doing it for themselves*. J Fam Plann Reprod Health Care 2009; 35:71–72). It probably works through being what might be termed a pharmacological curettage, after which with resumed Pill-taking oligo-amenorrhoea often returns and the need for such bleeding-triggered breaks usually gets less with time.

Drug interactions

Interacting drugs can reduce the efficacy of COCs by induction of liver enzymes, which leads to increased elimination of both estrogen and progestogen (Fig. 10). This effect can as much as halve blood levels of both hormones, and is clinically important (see below).

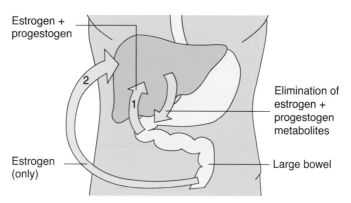

Figure 10
The enterohepatic recirculation of estrogen: (1) 'first pass'—absorption of hormones in the liver; (2) 'second pass'—reabsorption of active estrogen (not progestogen).

Do antibiotics matter any more?

In 2010, WHO reviewed the evidence relating to the recirculation of EE by mechanism 2 in Figure 10. This can potentially be impaired by antibiotics that reduce the population of certain gut flora that normally split estrogen metabolites. However, WHO found that any resulting lowering of EE levels is insufficient for any study to have proven either ovulation or conception as a consequence. *It seems this never was a real problem*! Presumably the many previous reports of COC failures because of antibiotics must have been primarily coincidental to missing tablets, which is certainly a common enough factor to coincide. Omissions might additionally occur through vomiting (due to the disease or antibiotic).

WHOMEC (and UKMEC) therefore *advise no restriction on use (WHO 1) of COCs, or more generally CHCs, if there is co-administration of antibiotics that are not enzyme inducers*—i.e. other than rifampicin/rifabutin—and therefore no extra precautions are now (2011) advised by the BNF as well as the FSRH.

However, they do recommend that women maintain meticulous Pill-taking during their illness and are advised about what to do if their antibiotic (or the illness) were to cause vomiting or severe diarrhoea.

Enzyme-inducing drugs

The most clinically important drugs with which this kind of interaction occurs are listed below.

The main clinically important enzyme-inducer drugs that might be co-administered with CHCs
• Rifampicin, rifabutin = the strongest
• Rufinamide
• Barbiturates
• Phenytoin
• Carbamazepine
• Oxcarbazepine
• Eslicarbazepine
• Primidone

- Topiramate (if daily dose >200 mg)
- Modafinil
- Aprepitant
- Some antiretrovirals (e.g. ritonavir, nevirapine)—full details are obtainable from www.hiv-druginteractions.org
- St John's Wort—potency of shop-bought product varies enormously; Committee on the Safety of Medicines (CSM) advises non-use with COC or POP

Clinical implications

Short-term use of an enzyme-inducing drug in a CHC-user—defined as <2 months

Recommended regimen
- Additional contraceptive precautions—usually condoms—are advised during the treatment, and should then be continued, since enzyme induction is sustained, for 28 days. A one-off shot of DMPA may be ideal (see below).
- If at the end of treatment there are fewer than seven tablets left in the pack (i.e. the third week), the next PFI should be eliminated (skip any placebo Pills).

Long-term use of enzyme inducers (except rifamycins)

This applies chiefly to epileptic women and women being treated for tuberculosis. This situation is WHO 3, meaning that an alternative method of contraception is preferable—especially for those on rifampicin or rifabutin, whose effects on the efficacy of CHCs are so strong that long-term users should use another method (WHO 4).

Better options that should always first be discussed are the injectable DMPA (with no special advice now needed to shorten the injection interval, see p. 93), an IUD or LNG-IUS. Implants are not advised (p. 107).

Except for the above WHO 4 drugs, if the woman insists on a COC:

Recommended regimen

- Prescribe an increased dose, usually 50 to 60 μg estrogen by taking two tablets daily, and also:
- Advise one of the extended use or tricycle regimens described above (this is particularly appropriate in epilepsy, since the frequency of attacks is often reduced by maintenance of more stable hormone levels), and *also*:
- If the COC is not taken 365/365, the user should be taught to shorten her PFI at the end of each tricycle: restarting after 4 days, even if the withdrawal bleed has not stopped.

Only one 50 μg Pill remains on the UK market (Table 2) and metabolic conversion of the prodrug mestranol to EE is only about 75% efficient. Therefore, Norinyl-1[TM] is almost identical to Norimin[TM]. So the FSRH recommends constructing a 50- or 60 μg regimen from two sub-50 μg products, e.g. two tablets daily of Microgynon 30, or e.g. as appropriate Femodene[TM] plus a Femodette[TM] tablet (see Table 2). As this practice is unlicensed, this is named-patient use and the guidance on pp. 173–175 should be followed. The woman can be reassured that she is metaphorically 'climbing a down escalator' so as to stay in the right place—her increased liver metabolism meaning that her body should still in reality be receiving a normal low-dose regimen.

Breakthrough bleeding and enzyme-inducer drugs

Breakthrough bleeding (BTB) may occur—indeed, it could have been the first clue to a drug interaction. If the long-term user of an enzyme inducer develops persistent BTB, the first step is to exclude another cause (see the checklist box on p. 63). Then recommend a 4- to 7-day break in the continuous tablet-taking. If the problem persists after restarting tablets, a change of method will nearly always be preferable.

The alternative of trying an even higher dose, combining Pills to a total estrogen content of maximum 70 μg in an attempt to increase the blood levels of both hormones to above the threshold for bleeding, is a possibility endorsed by the FSRH Drug Interactions guidance document (2011), but not ideal, given uncertainty about the VTE risk (despite the enzyme induction occurring).

Cessation of enzyme inducers after long-term use

It has been shown that 4 or more weeks may elapse before excretory function in the liver reverts to normal. Hence, if any of these drugs has been used for >1 month (or at all in the case of rifampicin/rifabutin), there should be a delay of about 4 weeks before returning to a standard low-dose regimen. This period should be increased to 8 weeks after more prolonged use of enzyme inducers. In all cases, there should be no PFI gap between the higher-dose and low-dose packets.

See also useful appendices to the FSRH guidance (URL on p. 59).

Drugs that do NOT pose a clinically important CHC efficacy problem

(despite appearing on past lists, e.g. based only on animal work)
  Griseofulvin
  Lansoprazole and other proton-pump inhibitors
  Ethosuximide
  Valproate
  Clonazepam
  Most newer anti-epileptic drugs not in box above

Other clinically relevant interacting drugs
Drugs whose own effects may be altered by the COC

- *Ciclosporin* levels can be *raised* by COC hormones: the risk of toxic effects means blood levels should be measured.

- *Potassium-sparing diuretics*: there is a risk of hyperkalaemia with drospirenone, the progestogen in Yasmin (or Yaz, p. 67), so these diuretics should not be used (WHO 4) with that COC.

- *Lamotrigine* levels can be *lowered* by CHCs, due to induction by EE of the enzyme glucuronyltransferase which eliminates the anti-epileptic through glucuronidation (see box).

Starting a COC in a patient stabilized on a regimen including lamotrigine risks causing an iatrogenic seizure through lowered levels
- This is WHO 3—any non-EE containing contraceptive would definitely be preferable (or a change of anti-epileptic regimen).

- Otherwise, seek her neurologist's advice re a pre-emptive increment in the dose of lamotrigine.
- There is logic in a continuous 365/365 regimen (as above) to prevent lamotrigine toxicity, which has been reported due to higher blood levels on the rebound in each PFI.
- *Exception*: If the woman is taking another enzyme inducer as well (since this will already have maximally induced the relevant enzyme) or valproate (which inhibits lamotrigine metabolism).
- There is also no problem in giving lamotrigine to patients already taking a COC, because the enzyme is already induced (as above): so the dose of anti-epileptic drug may as usual be titrated to the patient's needs.

The lamotrigine dose may need to be lowered when the COC is discontinued, or even during the PFI: hence ideal is 1st bullet of this box!

To date (2012), the available evidence supports EE within CHCs being the cause of lowered lamotrigine blood levels: so pending more data any progestogen-only alternative can be offered.

For more information visit:
www.fsrh.org/pdfs/CEUGuidanceDrugInteractionsHormonal.pdf

Counselling and ongoing supervision

Starting the COC

After taking a full personal and family history, with full consideration of possible contraindications on the WHO 1 to 4 scale, as described above, each woman deserves individual teaching, backed by the fpa's user-friendly leaflet *Your Guide to the Combined Pill* (as well as by the manufacturer's PIL).

After dealing with the woman's concerns and any questions she may have about risks and benefits—particularly about cancer and circulatory disease—and about 'minor' side effects, the recommended starting routines should be followed as in Table 7. Note the important footnotes.

Quick starting

Traditionally, 'medical' methods of contraception such as COCs have been scheduled always to start with or just after the woman's next menstrual period. As discussed on pp. 167–169, this policy is now seen in many cases as having been less than

Table 7
Starting routines for COCs

Condition	Start when?	Extra precautions for 7[a] days?
1 Menstruating	Day 1	No[b]—if starting with an active tablet
	Day 2	No[c]
	Day 3 or later	Yes
	Sunday start[b]	Yes, unless Sunday = day 1 or 2
	Any time in cycle ('Quick start')	Yes[d] and if reasonably sure not already conceived or at high conception risk (p. 166ff)
2 Post-partum a. No lactation	Day 21 (low risk of thrombosis by then[e], first ovulations reported day 28+)	No
b. Lactation	Not normally recommended at all (POP/injectable preferred)	
3 Post induced abortion/ miscarriage/ trophoblastic disease	Same day—or next day to avoid post-operative vomiting risk. Day 21 if was at/beyond 24 weeks' gestation	No, only needed if COC started >7 days later
4 Post higher-dose COC	Instant switch[f]—or use condoms for 7 days after the PFI	No
5 Post lower- or same-dose COC	After usual 7-day break, or instantly at choice	No
6 Post POP	First day of period	No
7 Post POP with secondary amenorrhoea, not pregnant	Any day (Sunday? Has advantages)	No
8 Post DMPA, implant, or IUD/IUS (risk of pregnancy excluded)	Any day (see text, usually ideal to overlap the new method with old)	No
9 Post IUD/IUS removal	Removed on day of starting COC	Yes, as ovulation still occurs with IUD/IUS
10 Other secondary amenorrhoea (risk of pregnancy excluded)	Any day (Sunday?)	Yes

Note that FSRH recommendations are slightly less cautious than mine, taking less account of risk of early ovulation in the first cycle.
[a]9 days for Qlaira (see text).
[b]ED Pill-users also start with the first active Pill on day 1. By applying the right sticky strip (out of seven supplied) for that weekday, all future Pills are then labelled with the correct days. A simpler alternative to explain is 'Sunday start', in which the woman delays taking the first active Pill till the first Sunday after her period starts, with condom use sustained through until seven active Pills have been taken (this also ensures that from then onwards there are no bleeds at weekends).
[c]Delay into day 2 can sometimes help, to be sure a period is normal, especially after EC.
[d]Immediate starts—'Quick starting'—means starting any day well beyond day 3 (i.e. not waiting as in past practice for that elusive *next* period) and are entirely acceptable, provided the prescriber is satisfied there has been no earlier conception or unacceptable conception risk in that cycle (see text here and at pp. 167–169). EC may sometimes be given first.
[e]Puerperal risk lasts longer after severe pregnancy-related hypertension, or the related HELLP syndrome (haemolysis, elevated liver enzymes, low platelets), so delay COC use until the return of normal BP and biochemistry. This history in the past is WHO 1.
[f]Perhaps too cautious: but if 7-day break taken, there are historical anecdotes of 'rebound ovulation' at the time of transfer.

ideal. If the provider can be 'reasonably sure' about absence of conception risk, it is now accepted, by WHO, UKMEC and other authorities, as entirely appropriate to advise a woman to start her COC or other medical method on the day she is first seen.

At any time, the user of contraception should be advised about maintaining sexual health. She should be warned, if now or at any future time she knows she is not in a mutually monogamous relationship, to use condoms (ideally supplied on site), in addition to the COC or other 'medical' method. The main take-home messages to be conveyed to a new user are summarized below.

Take-home messages for a new COC-taker

- Your fpa leaflet: this is not to be read and thrown away, it is something to keep safely in a drawer somewhere, for ongoing reference.
- The Pill only works if you take it correctly: if you do, each new pack will always start on the same day of the week.
- Even if bleeding, like a 'period', occurs (BTB), carry on Pill-taking: ring for advice if necessary. Nausea is another common early symptom. Both usually settle as your body gets used to the Pill.
- **Never be a late restarter of your Pill!** Even if your 'period' (withdrawal bleed) has not stopped yet, never start your next packet late. This is because the PFI is obviously a time when your contraceptive is not being supplied to your ovaries, so they might anyway be beginning to escape from its actions.
- Lovemaking during the 7 days after any packet is only safe if you do actually go on to the next pack. Otherwise (e.g. if you decide to stop the method) you must start using condoms after the last Pill in the pack.
- For what to do if any Pill(s) are more than 24 hours late (see p. 50).
- Other things that may stop the Pill from working include vomiting and some drugs (always mention that you are on the Pill).
- See a doctor at once if any of the things on p. 70 occur, especially new headaches with strange changes in your eyesight happening beforehand.
- As a one-off, you can shorten one PFI to make sure all your future withdrawal bleeds avoid weekends.
- You can avoid bleeding on holidays etc. by running packs together. (Discuss this with whoever provides your Pills, if you want to continue missing out 'periods' long term.)

- Good though it is as a contraceptive, the Pill does not give enough protection against *Chlamydia* and other STIs. Whenever in doubt, especially with a new partner, use a condom as well.
- Finally, always feel free to telephone or come back at any time (maybe to the practice nurse) for any reasons of your own, including any symptoms you would like dealt with.

NB Very similar advice applies also to users of the other CHCs: i.e. the patch or vaginal ring.

Second choice of Pill brand

How this relates to the symptom of breakthrough bleeding

Some women react unpredictably, and it is a false expectation that any single Pill will suit all women. Individual variations in motivation and tolerance of minor side effects are well recognized.

But, due to differences in absorption and metabolism, there is also marked variability (threefold, in the area under the curve) in blood levels of the exogenous hormones (Fig. 11).

This is relevant to the management of irregular bleeding.

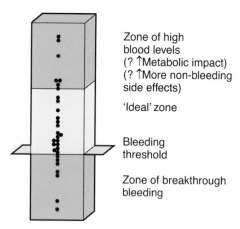

Figure 11
Schematic representation of the marked individual variation in blood levels of both contraceptive steroids.

Bleeding side effects

Given the 'model' shown in Figure 11 by the variability of blood levels and BTB risk, prescribers should try to identify the lowest dose for each woman that does not cause BTB. This should minimize adverse side effects, both serious and minor, and also reduce measurable metabolic changes. Since COCs all have a powerful contraceptive effect, this approach does not appear to impair effectiveness (far more important is not lengthening the PFI; see above). Even if BTB occurs, provided there is ongoing good Pill-taking, additional contraception is not needed.

The D-checklist for abnormal bleeding in a Pill-user

- **DISEASE:** Consider examining the cervix (it is not unknown for bleeding from an invasive cancer to be wrongly attributed, also a report of BTB should always trigger the thought: '*Chlamydia*?)'.
- **DISORDERS of PREGNANCY** that cause bleeding (e.g. retained products if the COC was started after a recent termination of pregnancy).
- **DEFAULT:** BTB may be triggered 2 or 3 days after a single missed Pills episode and may be persistent thereafter.
- **DRUGS,** if they are enzyme inducers (see text). Cigarettes are also drugs in this context: BTB has been shown to be statistically more common among smokers.
- **Diarrhoea** and/or **VOMITING:** Diarrhoea alone has to be exceptionally severe to impair absorption significantly.
- **DISTURBANCES of ABSORPTION:** For example, after massive gut resection (rare).
- **DURATION of USE too short:** BTB after starting on any new formulation may settle, if the pill-taker perseveres for 3 months. The opposite may apply during tricycling or other sustained use (see pp. 51–53), namely that the duration of continuous use has been too long for that woman's endometrium to be sustained, in which case a bleeding-triggered break may be taken (p. 54).
- **DOSE:** After the above have been excluded, it is possible to try
  – a phasic Pill if the woman is receiving monophasic treatment;
  – increasing first the progestogen then (maybe) the estrogen dose;
  – a different progestogen (some evidence that GSD, DSG and NGM give better cycle control than LNG Pills); or
  – NuvaRing, which produced less BTB and spotting in the first year of an RCT than Microgynon 30 (Oddsson, 2005, see Fig. 12).

Modified from Sapire E. Contraception and Sexuality in Health and Disease. New York: McGraw-Hill, 1990.

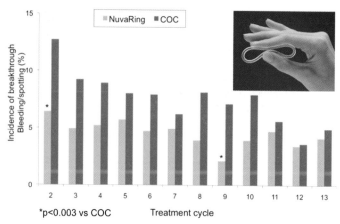

Figure 12

The incidence of breakthrough bleeding/spotting during cycles 2 to 13 in RCT (n = 1079) comparing NuvaRing with COC (Microgynon 30[TM]). Source: From Oddsson et al. Hum Reprod 2005; 20:557–562.

- The objective is that each woman should receive the least long-term metabolic impact that her uterus will allow, i.e. the lowest dose of contraceptive steroids that is just—but only just—above her bleeding threshold.
- If BTB does occur and is unacceptable or persists beyond two cycles, a different progestogen, or a higher dose may be tried, somewhat empirically: though only **after** the checks in the so-called 'D-checklist', see the Box above (p. 63).

Basically, it is vital first to exclude other causes of BTB, especially *D for Disease*, before blaming the COC!

Second choice of Pill if there are non-bleeding side effects

- When symptoms occur, it is generally bad practice to give further prescriptions to control them without changing the COC—such as diuretics for weight gain or antidepressants for mood symptoms.

- Aside from trying another CHC (NuvaRing?) or another method, there are two empirical courses of action for problems unrelated to bleeding—to decrease the dose of either hormone, if possible (estrogen can be avoided by trying a POP); or to use a different CHC progestogen.
- Additionally, although the evidence is anecdotal/empirical and there are almost no relevant RCTs, there is a little guidance available for side effects and conditions associated with a relative excess of either sex steroid (see boxes below).

Which second choice of Pill? Relative estrogen excess	
Symptoms	**Conditions**
<ul><li>Nausea</li><li>Dizziness</li><li>Leg cramps</li><li>Cyclical weight gain (fluid-related), 'bloating'—Yasmin is also worth a try here despite its estrogenicity, given the anti-mineralocorticoid activity of drospirenone</li><li>Vaginal discharge (no infection)</li><li>Some cases of breast enlargement attributed to fluid</li><li>Some cases of lost libido without depression, theoretically more likely if taking an anti-androgen (but no hard data)—as in Yasmin or Dianette and its generics</li></ul>	<ul><li>Benign breast disease</li><li>Fibroids</li><li>Endometriosis</li></ul>

For any of these try a progestogen-dominant COC, such as Microgynon 30.

Which second choice of Pill? Relative progestogen excess	
Symptoms	**Conditions**
<ul><li>Dryness of vagina</li><li>Depression/lassitude</li><li>Depressed mood ± associated loss of libido</li><li>Breast tenderness</li><li>*Anxiety about* weight gain—there is no good evidence that modern COCs cause the weight gain for which they are often blamed</li></ul>	<ul><li>Acne/seborrhoea</li><li>Hirsutism</li></ul>

Treat with estrogen-dominant COC such as Marvelon or, in moderately severe cases of acne or mild hirsutism, Yasmin or Dianette or its generics (see text). Caution is necessary in that estrogen dominance may correlate with a slightly higher risk of VTE, especially if high BMI (Table 5, pp. 30-32).

Why choose Yasmin™?

Acne, seborrhoea and sometimes hirsutism may be benefited by any of the estrogen-dominant COCs. Yasmin is a monophasic COC containing 3-mg DSP and 30 μg EE. DSP differs from other progestogens in COCs because:

- It acts as an anti-androgen, so the combination is an alternative to Dianette for the treatment of moderately severe acne and PCOS.
- It has diuretic properties due to anti-mineralocorticoid activity.

Yasmin is a useful choice for appropriate women, for example:

- A clear indication for estrogen/anti-androgen therapy, such as moderately severe acne (Marvelon works well for milder cases), including cases associated with PCOS.
- As a useful second choice for empirical control of minor side effects: particularly those associated with fluid retention such as bloatedness and cyclical breast enlargement. It seems to be of value for women with PMS, whether in their normal cycle or also occurring on another COC—in which case continuous use or tricycling is preferable.
- Last, and definitely least, what about weight? In one study, there was a maintained slight (about 1%) reduction of body mass, but most probably due to diuresis, hence less total body water compared with controls. Also, if the BMI is already above 30, there is a safety issue for this or any COC—although if it is being given for therapy, the risk-benefit analysis may be different (see p. 35).

What if a woman declares the COC is her only acceptable method and cannot be reassured about the weight gain issue, especially with a history of cyclical fluid retention–linked weight gain with previously used COCs? In my view, this would justify a trial of Yasmin (or Yaz™).

YAZ™

Available in some countries, Yaz delivers a lower daily dose of ethinylestradiol (20 μg) with drospirenone (p. 26) 3000 mg. Its 24/4 regimen with a 4-day Pill-free interval definitely increases efficacy (p. 51). While being an option among CHCs for any woman, these facts usually make Yaz—IF available—preferable to Yasmin (JG's view) for the special indications here: acne and severe PMS (known as premenstrual dysphoric disorder [PMDD] in the United States).

What now about Dianette™ (Clairette™/Acnocin™/ Cicafem™)?

This is another anti-androgen plus estrogen combination—co-cyprindiole, with cyproterone acetate (CPA) 2 mg plus EE 35 μg—licensed for the treatment of moderately severe acne and mild hirsutism in women. These are its indications, but practically everything about the COC in this book applies also to Dianette: it is a reliable anovulant, usually giving good cycle control, and has similar rules for missed tablets, interactions, absolute and relative contraindications, and requirements for monitoring.

RCT evidence shows that Yasmin has at least as good effectiveness for the conditions for which Dianette is indicated, and so might be used from the outset. Both are estrogen-dominant products requiring careful assessment of VTE risk factors. Given the apparent metabolic 'anti-estrogenicity' of LNG (p. 25), the expected relatively increased VTE risk compared with LNG Pills has now (2011) been shown for COCs using either DSP or CPA.

Duration of treatment with Dianette needs to be individualized. In the SPC (data sheet), it is recommended that treatment is withdrawn 3 to 4 months *after* the acne or hirsutism is completely resolved, but 'repeat courses may be given if the condition recurs'. In 2008 the MHRA confirmed this: '...co-cyprindiol can be re-started at any time if acne or hirsutism recurs on stopping treatment'.

Clinical implications

Unless there are strong grounds for continued use of Dianette rather than Yasmin (whose SPC mentions no duration limits), it is usual:

- to encourage patients to switch when their condition is controlled, see above, commonly to Marvelon™. The latter can be promoted to the woman as likely to be quite sufficient as maintenance treatment for what should now be well-controlled acne;
- if there is a relapse, to try Yasmin; or
- exceptionally, it may be appropriate to return to use of Dianette or a related generic (Table 2) for much longer.

When might one ever use Qlaira?

This COC contains estradiol valerate (hydrolysed in vivo to natural estradiol, E2) and dienogest, a moderately anti-androgenic progestogen. A complicated phasic regimen (four phases plus two lactose placebos, see Table 2) was unavoidable, because of using *natural* estrogen which is less potent than EE. With it, there is comparable cycle control to COCs using 20 μg EE. But users need warning about absent withdrawal bleeds in c. 20% of cycles.

Maintaining efficacy

There are only 2 days completely hormone-free plus 4 more days of E2-only, so the manufacturer advises slightly different rules for missed Pills which err very much on the side of caution. Simplified, these are as follows:

If an active tablet is forgotten for more than 12 hours, take it and the next when due + 9 (nine) *days extra precautions. In addition, for late omissions in the pack (days 18–24), discard the current wallet and restart new pack immediately the omission recognized*—so logically missing out the later days of reduced or absent hormones (see SPC). This advice may change with more experience: even now a 'missed Pill' could be more than 24 hours late, in my view. EC should be advised as well (JG's opinion), whenever enough early Pills in a pack have been missed to total more than 8 days in which *combined* hormones have not been taken and unprotected sexual intercourse (UPSI) also occurred.

Table 7 applies with the one difference that there should be 9 days of added precautions wherever the Table has '7 days'.

Metabolic effects

Using a less potent estrogen, with monthly total dosage slightly less than some hormone-replacement therapy (HRT) products, metabolic effects *seem* good (including low levels of D-dimer *suggesting* lowered intravascular thrombosis and fibrinolysis), but there is no epidemiological evidence, as yet, of fewer thrombotic events.

Stopping COCs

The first menstruation after stopping COCs (for any reason) is often delayed, but not usually for more than about 6 weeks. Secondary amenorrhoea for more than 6 months should always be investigated, whether or not it occurs after stopping COCs— the link will be coincidental and not causal. Whatever the diagnosis, any associated estrogen deficiency should not be allowed to continue long term without treatment.

Listed below are the (only) reasons for discontinuing COCs immediately or soon, and should be understood by all well-counselled women from their first visit (similar lists are in most PILs, and in the FPA's recommended leaflet *Your Guide to the Combined Pill*). The worst implications of these symptoms are Pill-related thrombotic or embolic catastrophes in the making.

Often there turns out to be another explanation for the symptom, and the COC may be recommenced later. Pending diagnosis, the COC, because of its contained EE, should be stopped, but any progestogen-only method (e.g. Cerazette) could be started immediately.

Symptoms for which COCs should be stopped immediately, pending investigation and treatment
- Unusual or severe and very prolonged headache
- Diagnosis of aura (see above), usually involving loss of part or whole of the field of vision on one side, with *or without* headache following
- Loss of sight in one eye (unassociated with migraine)
- Disturbance of speech (notably dysphasia in migraine with aura)
- Numbness, severe paraesthesia or weakness on one side of the body, e.g. one arm, side of the tongue; indeed, any symptom suggesting cerebral ischaemia or TIA
- A severe unexplained fainting attack or severe acute vertigo or ataxia
- Focal epilepsy
- Painful swelling in the calf
- Pain in the chest, especially pleuritic pain
- Breathlessness or cough with bloodstained sputum
- Severe abdominal pain
- Immobilization, for example
  – after most lower limb fractures, or
  – major surgery, or
  – leg surgery

In all the above circumstances, stop COC and consider anti-thrombotic treatment. If an elective procedure is planned and the Pill is stopped more than 2 weeks ahead (4 weeks is preferable), anti-coagulation is not usually necessary. Contraception can be maintained nowadays by switching to and then later from Cerazette, which is believed to have negligible prothrombotic effects.

Other reasons for early discontinuation:
- Acute jaundice
- BP >160/95 mmHg on repeated measurement (p. 41)
- Severe skin rash (erythema multiforme)
- Detection of a significant new risk factor or interacting disease, e.g. onset of severe SLE, first diagnosis of breast cancer

Pill follow-up: what is important?

Aside from the management of established risk factors or diseases already present, or that may suddenly or more gradually appear, and of new minor side effects (both dealt with above), follow-up primarily entails two items of monitoring:

- blood pressure and
- headaches, especially migraine.

Blood pressure

Monitoring of BP is vital. It should be recorded before COCs are started and checked after 3 months (1 month in a high-risk case) and subsequently at intervals of 6 months. COCs should always be stopped altogether if BP increase is entirely COC-related and exceeds 160/95 mmHg on repeated measurements (p. 38). A more moderate increase still suggests the possibility of an increased risk of arterial disease, especially in the presence of any other arterial risk factors (see Table 6).

However, if a COC-taker remains normotensive, with no rise between successive measurements during (in my view) the first year or so (UKMEC proposes this as soon as after the 3-month visit), annual follow-up of COC-users should now be the norm—in women without risk factors. This is good practice so long as it is made abundantly clear that they may return sooner for advice, as and when they may wish—a truly 'open-house' policy.

Headaches

Not to ask about a COC-taker's headaches at any regular or requested Pill follow-up visit would be a serious omission (see pp. 42–43 for the crucial importance of identifying migraine with aura and how to do it).

Screening

Note what is **not** included above in the follow-up requirements: neither breast and bimanual pelvic examinations nor monitoring blood tests have any relevance to Pill follow-up. Routine bimanual pelvic examinations in asymptomatic COC-takers are particularly uncalled for, because the disorders causing detectable pelvic masses or tenderness are all actually less frequent in COC-takers than in others, as listed on p. 15.

Even taking cervical smears is for screening and not primarily a COC-associated exercise. After the age of 25, cervical screening should simply be performed regularly, as guidelines recommend for all sexually active women.

Congenital abnormalities and fertility issues

Any possible effect of COCs on congenital abnormalities is hard to establish because it is so difficult to prove a negative; moreover, 2% of all full-term fetuses have a significant malformation.

- Even with exposure during organogenesis, meta-analyses of the major studies fail to show an increased risk. If present, it must be very small.
- Used prior to the conception cycle, the conclusions of a WHO scientific group have not since been challenged—namely, that there is no good evidence for any adverse effects on the fetus of COCs. It can do no harm if a woman stops COCs and switches to barriers for 2 or more months before conception, but there is no objective evidence that it is worth the effort. Certainly, any woman who finds herself pregnant immediately after stopping COCs should be strongly reassured.

What about 'taking breaks' to optimize fertility?

Concerns about its reversibility have dogged the COC since its first marketing. Fertile ovulation can be minimally delayed on cessation, for a matter of days or up to 4 weeks—a much shorter time than following injectable use (see below). Yet, just as for the latter method, there is no evidence that COCs can cause permanent loss of fertility. Indeed, a large study (Hum Reprod 2002; 17:2754–2761) showed that use of the COC for more than 5 years before the 8497 planned conceptions was associated with a decreased risk of delay in conceiving.

If a woman still feels more comfortable to take a routine break from the COC, we should always help her to find a satisfactory contraceptive alternative. However, there is no known benefit to

- fertility or
- health

from taking short elective breaks of 6 months or so every few years, as was once recommended.

In one study, a quarter of young women who took breaks as above had unwanted conceptions. Relevantly, another finding of the Human Reproduction report quoted above was that one-third of the whole population admitted their pregnancy was not truly planned—and this was a large population surveyed in antenatal clinics, and thus could not include those who had pregnancies terminated.

Summary
- The first visit for prescription of COCs is by far the most important, and should never be rushed. A second visit in the first week, to the same or maybe a different provider in the surgery, provides a valuable opportunity for questions.
- The LARCs, long-term and 'forgettable' contraceptive options should always be included in the discussion, despite the woman's presenting request for what she happens to know about (most probably the Pill).
- If the Pill remains her choice, along with discussing the risks and benefits, and fully assessing her medical and family history—all at her level of understanding—there is much ground to cover (see the 'Take-home messages' list above). Often it is useful to share this between the doctor and practice or clinic nurse.
- Thereafter, there are really only three key components to COC monitoring during follow-up:
  – BP
  – Headaches
  – Identification and management of any new risk factors/diseases/side effects

No matter how carefully those with contraindications are excluded, a few women will experience adverse effects. Repeated presentation with multiple side effects sometimes suggests the offer of a different method rather than a different Pill—or, that a psychosexual problem needs to be faced.

For more, including most references for this chapter, visit: www. fsrh.org/pdfs/CEUGuidanceCombinedHormonalContraception.pdf

TRANSDERMAL COMBINED HORMONAL CONTRACEPTION: EVRA™

Evra is a transdermal patch delivering EE with norelgestromin, the active metabolite of NGM. The daily skin dose of 33.9 μg EE with 203 μg norelgestromin is intended to produce blood levels in the reference range of those after a tablet of Cilest but without either the diurnal fluctuations or the oral peak dose given to the liver.

Pending more data, all the absolute and relative contraindications and indeed most of the above practical management advices in chapters 5 and 6 about the COC apply to this CHC, with obvious minor adjustments. It can be seen as a bit like 'Cilest through the skin'.

However, in the United States, the FDA requires a warning in the Evra SPC, initially based on its pharmacokinetics, that patch-users are exposed to about 60% more total estrogen; moreover, two out of three case-control studies show an increased risk of VTE, compared with oral COCs with 30 to 35 μg estrogen. In other studies, Evra also produced relatively more estrogen-associated side effects such as breast tenderness and nausea. The FDA concluded (2008) that 'Ortho Evra is a safe and effective method of contraception when used according to the labelling' but advises added caution for women with VTE risk factors.

In studies, the patch had excellent adhesion even in hot climates and when bathing or showering; the incidence of detachment of patches was 1.8% (complete) and 2.9% (partial). About 2% of women had local skin reactions which led to discontinuation. In the pooled analysis of three pivotal studies [Fertility and Sterility 2002; (2 suppl 2)], the Pearl index for consistent users of Evra was similar to that for oral Pills—and less than 1 per 100 woman-years.

Interestingly, in the clinical trials, one-third of the few failures occurred in the 3% weighing above 90 kg. In my view, this apparently reduced effectiveness contraindicates (WHO 4) Evra for such women, when added to the VTE risk from the BMI they are likely to have weighing 90 kg, anyway. They are far from ideal users of this estrogen-dominant product.

> **Maintenance of efficacy of Evra**
> - Avoid use at all if body weight >90 kg, indeed in all cases with a risk factor for VTE—on safety as well as efficacy grounds.
> - Warn the user that the contraceptive is in the glue of the patch, so a dry patch that has fallen off should not be re-used!
> - Each patch is worn for 7 days, for 3 consecutive weeks followed by a patch-free week. This regimen was shown to aid compliance, particularly in young women. Under age 20, 'perfect use' was reported in 68% of COC cycles, but 88% of patch cycles. Clinically, the patch, along with NuvaRing below, is therefore an alternative to offer to those who, refusing a LARC, find it difficult to remember a daily Pill. Usefully, there is a 2-day margin for error for late patch change. Setting up a weekly mobile text-reminder 'Today is your new patch day' can also help.
> - As with the COC, it is essential never to lengthen the contraception-free (patch-free) interval.
> - If this interval exceeds 8 days for any reason (either through late application or through the first new patch detaching and this being identified late), advise extra precautions for the duration of the first freshly applied patch (i.e. for 7 days). EC should be considered if there has been sexual exposure during the preceding patch-free time, if that exceeded 9 days.
> - Absorption problems through vomiting/diarrhoea have no effect on this method's efficacy, but:
> - During short-term enzyme-inducer therapy, and for 28 days after this ends, additional contraception (e.g. with condoms) is advised, plus elimination of any patch-free intervals during this time. For long-term therapy, advise another method: use of two patches at a time is not advised (UKMEC).

TRANSVAGINAL COMBINED HORMONAL CONTRACEPTION: NUVARING™

NuvaRing is a combined vaginal ring depicted in Figure 12 (p. 64) that releases etonogestrel (3-ketodesogestrel) 120 µg and EE 15 µg/day, thus equating to some degree with 'vaginal Mercilon'. It is normally retained for 3 weeks and then removed for a withdrawal bleed during the fourth week.

There is an option to remove it for up to 3 hours during sex, with extra precautions advised only if it is absent for longer.

Expulsion is uncommon, occurring usually in parous women, in only 2.3% in the first 13 cycles of a trial, of which 1.7% in the first 3 cycles (N = 3333). Instruction to users is just to wash it and reinsert, this rarely means they must change method.

Pending more dedicated information, all the absolute and relative contraindications, and most of the above practical management advice about the COC, apply also to this CHC. It appears to have a side-effect profile very like that of Mercilon itself.

In studies, it proved very popular, with maintained sexual satisfaction, excellent cycle control (see Fig. 12, p. 64) and a failure rate comparable to oral COCs.

It was also found (Contraception 2006; 73:488–492) that 'baseline discomfort with genital touching' was not a problem and could even be linked to high ring satisfaction.

Maintenance of efficacy of NuvaRing

- Expulsions were primarily during the emptying of bowels or bladder, and therefore readily recognized.
- As with the COC, it remains essential never to lengthen the contraception-free (ring-free) interval. If for any reason this exceeds 8 days, advise extra precautions for 7 days. As for Evra, EC should be considered if there has been sexual exposure during any ring-free time that exceeds 9 days.
- Advise as routine a day 28 ring-insertion reminder by mobile phone!
- Also, since ring when in situ is imperceptible to the user, the suggestion to make it part of foreplay to check it is there before sex might prevent some failures.
- Absorption problems and vomiting/diarrhoea have no detectable effect on this method's efficacy.
- During short-term enzyme-inducer therapy and afterwards for 28 days, additional contraception is advised, plus elimination of any ring-free intervals. For long-term therapy, advise another method.

Comparison between ring and patch—the ring seems to have the edge	
Ring	**Patch**
EE blood levels—Area under the curve lower: • 3.4 × in ring-users cpd with patch • 2.1 × cpd with COC	EE blood levels higher by 60% compared to 35 μg norgestimate COC
Less nausea and breast tenderness than patch or an EE-dominant COC So ring better choice if high BMI	Confirms patch is more estrogenic Method best avoided if VTE risk Also risk of failure in obesity (see text)
Expulsions occur (see text—continuation usually possible)	Patches can fall off
Vaginal symptoms reported more with ring. Not thrush or STIs. (? Lowered threshold to report?)	Skin reactions can cause discontinuation
In United States, RCT recruiting from COC-users, 71% ring-users vs. 27% patch-users wished to go on using, rather than return to COC (Creinin et al. Obstet Gynecol 2008)	
Better cycle control than 30 μg LNG-COC (see Fig. 12, p. 64)	

Note: These methods *share* an absorption advantage, if there is concern about reduced COC absorption in the upper small bowel such as in severe Crohn's disease (p. 40).

ZOELY™ — a new COC (2012) with natural estrogen, but monophasic

Available in some markets—not yet in the UK—this consists of 24 white active tablets each containing 2.5 mg nomegestrol acetate and 1.5 mg estradiol (as hemihydrate) with 4 yellow placebo tablets, hence sharing with Qlaira (p. 68) the advantage of a shortened PFI. Its progestogen is likewise potent, with moderately anti-androgenic activity. The total dose of estradiol per 28 days is 36 mg, which is less than in some marketed HRT products (cf. 56 mg in Kliofem™ or Nuvelle™). Pending more data Zoely, though not studied yet other than for contraception, hence appears to me, like Qlaira, as *contraceptive HRT* and so usable unlicensed (pp. 171–5) by otherwise risk factor–free older women until the menopause. The other special indications on p. 69 also apply, though only Qlaira has so far been licensed for HMB. Both are effective contraceptives, options for any sexually active women, and they usually provide good cycle control. Zoely has simpler monophasic packaging with the same advice for missed pills as for COCs using EE.

Progestogen-only pill

There are five varieties of progestogen-only Pill (POP) available (Table 8): four are of the old type that variably inhibit ovulation, while the fifth, Cerazette™, is a primarily anovulant product. Unless otherwise stated, the abbreviation POP will refer to the four old-type POPs. The latest Faculty Guidance on POPs can be accessed at www.fsrh.org/pdfs/CEUGuidanceProgestogenOnlyPill09.pdf, wherein the references to studies mentioned here can be found.

Table 8
Available POPs

Product	Constituents	Course of treatment
Noriday	350 µg norethisterone	28 tablets
Micronor	350 µg norethisterone	28 tablets
Femulen	500 µg etynodiol diacetate	28 tablets
Norgeston	30 µg levonorgestrel	35 tablets
Cerazette	75 µg desogestrel	28 tablets

MECHANISM OF ACTION AND MAINTENANCE OF EFFECTIVENESS

The mechanism of action is complex because of variable interactions between the administered progestogen and the endogenous activity of the woman's ovary. Outside of lactation (when their effectiveness is hugely enhanced, see below), fertile ovulation is prevented in 50% to 60% of cycles. In the remainder, there is reliance mainly on progestogenic interference with mucus penetrability. This 'barrier' effect is readily lost, so that each old-type POP tablet must be taken within 3 hours of the same regular time.

If POPs are indeed taken regularly each day within that time span of 27 hours, without breaks and regardless of bleeding patterns, they are in practice as effective (or as ineffective, in 'typical use, see Table 1!) as COCs—especially for those aged 35 and over.

Effectiveness

In the United Kingdom, the Oxford/FPA study reported a failure rate for old-tye POPs of 3.1 per 100 woman-years between the ages 25 and 29, but this improved to 1.0 at 35 to 39 years of age and was as low as 0.3 for women over 40 years of age. Realistically, most users are probably not as meticulous as those married middle-class women.

Cerazette is very different because it blocks ovulation in 97% of cycles and had a failure rate in the pre-marketing study of only 0.17 per 100 woman-years (in consistent users even without breastfeeding).

With regard to effect of body mass (not BMI), studies are suggestive, but not conclusive, that the failure rate of old-type POPs may be higher with increasing weight, as was well established in early studies of progestogen rings and some implants. Pending more data, a logical policy now is to make Cerazette one's first choice for women over 70 kg (irrespective of height), especially if they are young. This is preferable to taking two POPs, though that is still an option off-licence.

However, because of reduced fertility, there can be little doubt that one old-type POP daily will be adequately effective in older overweight women, above the age of 45, or during established breastfeeding.

Missed Pills

Loss of full contraceptive activity through missed Pills or vomiting (without successful replacement of the vomited tablet) is believed to start within as little as 3 hours, or 12 hours for Cerazette, but is corrected adequately (as far as the mucus is concerned) if renewed Pill-taking is combined with extra precautions for just 48 hours (UKMEC).

Clinically, after missing a POP for more than 3 hours (or more than 12 hours for Cerazette; see below) the woman should:
- take that day's Pill immediately and the next one on time
- use added precautions for the next 2 days

Additionally, with old-type POPs, if there has already been intercourse without added protection between the time of first potential loss of the mucus effect through to its restoration by 48 hours, it is appropriate to:
- advise immediate emergency contraception (EC) usually with levonorgestrel (see p. 149), with the next old-type POP being taken on time

What EC action is needed during full lactation taking ordinary POPs, or for Cerazette-users (who rely less on the mucus effect and have *at least* 12 hours of 'leeway' anyway?)

Here there is established anovulation (moreover without there being any of the COC's Pill-free intervals, with their contraception-weakening effect). So although the first two bullets above would apply, EC would be needed less often than implied in the above box—i.e. not in the majority of cases.

LACTATION AND THE POP

According to the lactational amenorrhoea method (LAM—see Fig. 20), even without the POP, there is only about a 2% conception risk if all three LAM criteria continue to apply.

LAM criteria
- Amenorrhoea, since the lochia ceased
- Full lactation—the baby's nutrition is effectively all from its mother
- Baby not yet 6 months old

This is why, on *any* POP (old-type or Cerazette) during full lactation, EC is very rarely indicated for missed POPs. But because breastfeeding varies in its intensity, if an old-type POP tablet is 3 hours late it is still usual to advise additional precautions during the next two tablet-taking days.

What dose to the baby?

During lactation, with all POPs (including Cerazette), the dose to the infant is believed to be harmless, but this aspect must always be discussed. The least amount of administered progestogen gets into the breast milk if the highly protein-bound LNG POP (Norgeston) is used. The quantity has been calculated to be the equivalent of one POP in 2 years—considerably less than the progesterone of cow's milk origin found in formula feeds.

If EC is required (exceptionally, see above, perhaps because of multiple Pill omissions) by a breastfeeding mother, once again very little LNG reaches the breast milk. She may wish to express and discard her breast milk for 8 to 12 hours, the dose reaching her baby becoming negligible thereafter.

Weaning

Beware—unwanted conceptions are common when lactating POP-users have not been adequately warned that their margin for error in POP-taking will diminish at weaning. This is one reason for using Cerazette, to maintain efficacy as lactational infertility wanes. Users of other POPs should be given a supply of a 'stronger' method, such as the COC or Cerazette, along with clear instructions to start it when breast milk stops being their baby's main nutrition, or no later than the first bleed.

Drug interactions

A reminder, **broad-spectrum antibiotics** do not interfere with the effectiveness of any hormonal method.

- **Enzyme inducers.** Another contraceptive method is advised during use of liver enzyme-inducers such as rifampicin or carbamazepine and continuing after stopping for at least 4 weeks (see above re COCs, pp. 55–6). Long-term treatment with enzyme inducers is WHO 3. But if a suitable alternative contraceptive is not identified and the couple do not wish to use condoms indefinitely, increasing the dose is an option (my view, not UKMEC)—usually to two Cerazettes daily, after assessing all relevant factors including lactation and the woman's body weight, age and likely fertility. This is unlicensed use (pp. 173–5).

- **Bosentan.** This endothelin antagonist is an enzyme-inducer drug that would never be relevant for any CHC, since it is used to treat pulmonary hypertension (which is WHO 4 for CHCs). However, Cerazette could be an option for a young woman with this serious condition—again with two tablets (my view, not UKMEC) being taken daily to compensate for the enzyme induction. Double-dosing use is always unlicensed.

Note: Better than above unlicensed double-dosing, especially as pregnancy can be lethal in pulmonary hypertension, would be the use of DMPA or an IUD or IUS, which are always preferred contraceptives where there is enzyme induction (p. 56).

ADVANTAGES

Healthwise, being EE-free, these are exceptionally safe products. There are negligible changes to most metabolic variables. There is no proven causative link

- with any tumour (there was a non-significant increase in breast cancer risk in the 1996 Collaborative Group Study (p. 17), which has not been confirmed)
- with venous or arterial disease
- with osteopenia, weight gain, depression or headache

INDICATIONS

See the box below for these. Some of them are WHO 2 not 1, but that always means "broadly usable": hence being an *indication* if a Pill-method is wanted and a COC would be WHO 3 or 4:

Indications for POP or Cerazette use
- Woman's choice—especially Cerazette. This should not now be seen as a 'second-choice' method, for use only when a COC is contraindicated or unacceptable
- Lactation, where the combination even with ordinary POPs is extra-effective—indeed as good as the COC would be in non-breastfeeders
- Side effects with, or recognized contraindications to, the combined Pill, in particular where estrogen-related. As EE-free products do not appear to significantly affect blood-clotting

mechanisms, POPs may be used (WHO 2) by women with a definite past history of VTE and a whole range of disorders predisposing to both arterial and venous disease (WHO 2). Good counselling and record-keeping are essential
- Major or leg surgery or over the time of treatments for varicose veins—when COCs are often contraindicated on VTE grounds (WHO 2)
- Sickle cell disease, severe structural heart disease, pulmonary hypertension (Cerazette preferred POP on efficacy grounds)
- Smokers above 35 years of age
- Hypertension, whether COC-related or not, controlled on treatment
- Migraine, including varieties with aura (WHO 2: the woman may well continue to suffer migraines, but the fear of an EE-promoted thrombotic stroke is eliminated). Cerazette is preferred, to obtain optimum stability of endogenous hormones whose fluctuation may cause attacks
- Diabetes mellitus (DM)—but caution WHO 3 if there is significant DM with tissue damage (see below)
- Obesity—but then usually prescribing Cerazette (see text)

Old-type POPs are still good during lactation and for the older woman, given diminished fertility; but for the young highly fertile woman, Cerazette is now the POP of choice.

RISKS AND DISADVANTAGES
Side effects

The main side effect of POPs and Cerazette is irregular bleeding, about which all prospective users should be clearly warned.

The irregularity can include oligo-amenorrhoea. This occurs more commonly with Cerazette than with other POPs. But, reassuringly, it appears that with all POPs, Cerazette and Nexplanon^{TM}, follicle-stimulating hormone (FSH) is not completely suppressed even during the amenorrhoea, which is mainly caused by luteinizing hormone (LH) suppression. There is therefore enough follicular activity at the ovary to maintain adequate mid-follicular phase estrogen levels. Pending more data, this means that there is not the concern about bone density reduction that exists for DMPA (see below).

For management of side effects during follow-up, see below.

CONTRAINDICATIONS

Absolute contraindications (WHO 4) for POP and Cerazette use

- Any serious adverse effect of CHCs not certainly related solely to the estrogen (e.g. *liver adenoma or cancer*, although UKMEC says UKMEC 3)
- Recent *breast cancer* not yet clearly in remission (see below)
- *Hypersensitivity to any component*
- Current *pregnancy*

WHO 3 conditions for POP and Cerazette use

- Current ischaemic heart disease, *severe arterial diseases* including stroke
- Sex-steroid-dependent cancer, including *breast cancer,* when in complete remission (UKMEC states UKMEC 4 until 5 years, then UKMEC 3). Agreement of the relevant hospital consultant should be obtained and the woman's autonomy respected: record that she understands it is unknown whether progestogen might alter the recurrence risk (either way)
- *Severe liver disease* (acute viral hepatitis, decompensated cirrhosis)
- *Acute porphyria*, if there is a history of actual attack triggered by hormones (my view, since progestogens as well as estrogens are believed capable of precipitating these attacks and 1% are fatal). Otherwise the history of acute porphyria is WHO 2 for all POPs
- Previous treatment for *ectopic pregnancy in a nulliparous woman*; however, this is an indication for Cerazette! The overall risk of recurrent ectopic pregnancy is reduced somewhat among old-type POP-users, which is why the condition is actually classified by UKMEC as UKMEC 1. But in my view it would be much better here to offer the COC, DMPA, Cerazette or Nexplanon than a POP, since the risk can be reduced still further by methods that regularly block fertilization—to better preserve the precious remaining fallopian tube
- Undiagnosed *genital tract bleeding* until cause established
- *Enzyme inducers*: although in my view two POPs can be taken, off-licence (see above), another method such as an injectable, IUD or LNG-IUS would again be preferable

There remain some conditions where the POP method is generally WHO 2. These as we have seen may sometimes be indications when other effective alternatives are rejected:

Weak relative contraindications (WHO 2) for POP and Cerazette use

- *Past VTE* or marked risk factors/*predispositions to VTE*
- *Risk factors for arterial disease* or current high risk including diabetes with arteriopathy; hypertension: more than one risk factor can be present, in contrast to CHCs
- Strong *family history of breast cancer*—UKMEC says UKMEC 1 for this
- *Known BRCA mutation* present
- *Current liver disorder*—even if there is persistent biochemical change—including compensated cirrhosis, history of CHC-related cholestasis
- *Gall bladder disease*
- Most other *chronic severe systemic diseases* including inflammatory bowel disease (but WHO 3 if there is known significant malabsorption of sex steroids)
- Past *symptomatic (painful) functional ovarian cysts.* But persistent cysts/follicles that are commonly detected on routine ultrasonography can be disregarded if they cause no symptoms. If desired, with this history Cerazette would be preferred to an old-type POP.
- Unwillingness to cope with prospect of irregularity or absence of periods—sometimes connected with cultural/religious taboos

COUNSELLING AND ONGOING SUPERVISION

The starting routines are summarized in Table 9. Crucial aspects of counselling are as follows:

- Clarity for prior COC-users that they should not take a 7-day break after 21 days! Every year because of the lack of this there occur what can only be termed 'iatrogenic' conceptions.
- Even more than for COCs, giving the most useful tip to dedicate one mobile phone alarm/text message to 'POP-taking time'.

Table 9
Starting routines for POPs

Condition before start	Start when?	Extra precautions?
Menstruation	Day 1 of period	No
	Days 2–5	No
	Any time in cycle ('Quick start')	2 days[a]
Post-partum		
No lactation	Usually day 21 (can be earlier)	No
Lactation	Day 21—maybe later if 100% lactation (UKMEC recommends) delay till 6 weeks)	No
After induced abortion/miscarriage	Same day	No
After COCs	Instant switch	No
Amenorrhoea (e.g. post-partum)	Any time[b]	2 days

[a]Can start any day in selected cases **if** the prescriber is satisfied there has been negligible conception risk up to the starting day.
[b]If pregnancy test negative, no recent high conception risk and follow-up arranged. POPs are not thought to be teratogenic. See pp. 167–9.

Frequent or prolonged menstrual bleeding

This is the main nuisance side effect. With advance warning, it may be tolerated. Improvement appears more likely with Cerazette, based on the randomized controlled trial comparing it with an LNG POP. By 1 year, around half of ongoing Cerazette-users reported amenorrhoea (which with counselling can be accepted as an advantage) or infrequent bleeding (one or two bleeds per 90 days).

But in this pre-market study, the improved bleeding pattern was only evident when users persevered beyond 6 months, and there is no treatment for prolonged or heavy bleeding that is reliably effective. Having excluded a coincidental cause (based on the D-checklist on p. 63), taking two tablets daily can be successful, anecdotally, often enough in my view to be worth a trial. Otherwise, the best bets are a change of POP or a change of method.

Amenorrhoea

Except during full lactation, prolonged spells of amenorrhoea occur most often in older women. Once pregnancy has been excluded, the amenorrhoea must be the result of anovulation, and so signifies very high efficacy—as well as convenience for many without evidence of harm.

Non-bleeding side effects

These are rare with POPs, apart from the following complaints:

- *Breast tenderness*, though common, is usually transient; if it recurs, it can sometimes be overcome by changing POPs—especially to Cerazette.
- *Functional cysts* or luteinized unruptured follicles are also not uncommon; however, most are symptomless, and pelvic pain on one or other side is relatively unusual.

Clinically, if functional cysts among POP-users do become symptomatic, they can lead to problems in the differential diagnosis from ectopic pregnancy (pain, menstrual disturbance and a tender adnexal mass being present in both conditions).

Monitoring

The BP of all POP-takers is checked initially, but thereafter if not raised it does not need to be taken more often than for other women. POP-takers need no regular visits—just the usual 'open-house' policy, the freedom to discuss *any* problems on request. If the BP was raised during COC use, it usually reverts to normal on POPs. If it does not, indeed, the woman most probably has essential hypertension.

Return of fertility after discontinuing POPs, including Cerazette

This is rapid: indeed clinically, from the user's point of view, fertility after stopping must be assumed to be immediate.

Menopause

Establishing ovarian failure at the menopause is less important than with CHCs, since all the POPs are safe enough products to continue using well into the sixth decade, usually in fact to age 55 when loss of fertility is almost invariable, as discussed later (p. 171). First switching to any POP from any other hormonal method, and then continuing till age 55, can be a reassuring way to manage that often difficult transition out of the reproductive years.

On an old-type POP (not the pituitary-suppressing Cerazette), if amenorrhoea and vasomotor symptoms appear above the age of 50, a high blood FSH measurement (>30 IU/L) suggests ovarian failure. This may then be confirmed by following Plan C on page 172.

However, if the FSH is found to be low, this suggests (despite the amenorrhoea) continuing ovarian function. If the POP is not simply continued to that age of 55 when ovarian function must be negligible, there would be need for continuing use of another contraceptive until then.

CERAZETTE

Mechanism of action and maintenance of effectiveness

This product contains 75 μg desogestrel and to some extent 'rewrites the textbooks' about POPs—mainly because it blocks ovulation in 97% of cycles and had a failure rate in the pre-marketing study of only 0.17 per 100 woman-years (and that without also breastfeeding). This makes it somewhat like 'Nexplanon by mouth'.

Following a reassuring European study, in which Cerazette tablets were deliberately taken late, 12 hours of 'leeway' in Pill-taking have been approved before extra precautions are advised—these then being for 2 days, as for other POPs (although the manufacturer's SPC still recommends 7 days). This has led in recent years to a surge in its popularity among young and highly fertile users for whom we would previously not even have suggested a POP.

Otherwise, Cerazette shares the medical safety and rapid reversibility—but also, unfortunately, the tendency to irregular bleeding side effects and functional ovarian cyst formation—of the old-type POPs.

Starting routines

See Table 9 (i.e. as other POPs). 'Missed Pills' advice is on p. 80.

Special indications (but no necessity for such, woman's choice is quite sufficient!)

- For a start, Cerazette is obviously free of all the risks attributable to EE; in addition, no effects on BP have been reported. Hence, it greatly broadens the indications for a progestogen-only method, in many cases where a CHC is WHO 4 or 3, but a Pill method with greater efficacy than ordinary POPs is desired.

- Cerazette is now a good option for many young fertile women with complicated *structural heart disease* or pulmonary hypertension (see above); or undergoing major or leg surgery.

- Given the earlier discussion about POPs and *body mass*, Cerazette would now be the first-choice POP for a woman weighing over 70 kg—taking the normal dose—unless she was breastfeeding or over 45 years of age, in which case any POP in normal daily dose would be effective.

- There are anecdotes of failure in good Cerazette-takers weighing >100 kg; and there is no expectation of harm if such unusually heavy women therefore choose after counselling to take 2 tablets a day (unlicensed use pp. 173–5).

- Cerazette also usually ablates the menstrual cycle like CHCs do, but without using EE. So it has potentially beneficial effects and can be tried (but not always successfully—no promises possible) in a range of disorders, including
  - past history of ectopic pregnancy (discussed above),
  - dysmenorrhoea,
  - menorrhagia,
  - mittelschmerz,
  - premenstrual syndrome (PMS).

Problems and disadvantages

As with all progestogen-only methods, irregular bleeding remains a very real problem. Indeed, this is the one area showing no great advantage in the pre-marketing comparative study with LNG 30-μg POP-users. The dropout rate for changes in bleeding pattern showed no difference, but among those who persevered, there was a useful trend for the more annoying frequent and prolonged bleeding experiences to lessen with continued use.

Despite this higher incidence of (more acceptable) oligo-amenorrhoea than with existing POPs, Cerazette (like other POPs and Nexplanon) appears to continue to provide adequate follicular phase levels of estradiol for bone health (p. 113).

Contraindications

These, whether WHO 4, 3 or 2, are very similar to those for old-type POPs listed above. The main difference is that Cerazette is more effective, making it positively suitable for a past history of ectopic pregnancy.

> **In summary:**
> Cerazette has now become a first-line hormonal contraceptive for many women. However, there is no strong indication to use it in full lactation or for older women above 45 years of age. One cannot expect to improve upon 100% contraception, which these two states do (almost) provide when combined with an old-type POP.

Injectables

BACKGROUND

In the United Kingdom, the only injectable currently licensed for long-term use is depot medroxyprogesterone acetate (DMPA)—Depo-Provera™.

Despite early campaigns against its use, this has been repeatedly endorsed by the expert committees of prestigious bodies, such as the International Planned Parenthood Federation (IPPF) and WHO. DMPA is without doubt even safer than COCs. WHO data indicate that DMPA-users have a reduced risk of cancer, with no overall increased risk of cancers of the breast, ovary or cervix—and a fivefold reduction in the risk of carcinoma of the endometrium (relative risk 0.2). There is still the possibility of a weak cofactor effect on breast cancer in current users, similar to that with COCs. However, this is unproven, and the apparent association in the early years of use may be due to surveillance bias.

Heffron et al (*Lancet Infectious Diseases* pub. on-line 4 Oct 2011) reinforced another concern, that HIV transmission is increased by DMPA. Yet causation remains uncertain: higher coital frequency and less condom use by DMPA-users are likely. WHO's 2012 review and resulting advice are awaited.

ADMINISTRATION

There are actually two injectable agents available: DMPA 150 mg every 12 weeks, and NET-EN (norethisterone enantate) Noris-terat™ 200 mg every 8 weeks. After well shaking the pre-loaded syringe for the former and pre-warming the ampoule for the latter which is oily, each is given by deep intramuscular injection in the first 5 days of the menstrual cycle. Injections may also be given well beyond day 5, with 7 days added precautions, if it is sufficiently certain that a conception risk has not been taken (p. 166). The injection sites, in the United Kingdom usually in the upper outer quadrant of either buttock, though the upper outer thigh and deltoid are also acceptable sites, should not be massaged.

Noristerat is not licensed for long-term contraception, though it can be so used off-licence (pp. 173–5), and will not be considered further here.

Subcutaneous DMPA

There is interest in this different route of administration, under the skin of the abdominal wall or upper thigh. The US marketed product is termed depo-subQ provera 104. It delivers a lower dose of medroxyprogesterone acetate (104 mg) than standard Depo-Provera for a similar duration of effectiveness. It was licensed in 2005 for the United Kingdom but is disappointingly still (2012) not available.

For developing countries, work is in progress to provide it in the Uniject™ system www.path.org/uniject.php. This is a small bubble of clear plastic pre-filled with a single dose and attached to a needle for one-time use. It is virtually impossible to re-use (e.g. by substance-abusers). Self-injection should be easy to teach and the end product could be supplied a year at a time, for administration to self—or to friends by each other.

MECHANISM OF ACTION AND EFFECTIVENESS

DMPA is one of the most effective among reversible methods (Table 1), with a 'perfect use' failure rate of 0.3 (3 in 1000) in the first year of use (Table 1). It functions primarily by causing anovulation, backed by similar effects on the cervical mucus to the POP/COC, as backup. A high initial blood level is achieved, declining over the next 3 months but staying above the level to inhibit ovulation for much longer in some women.

Potential drug interactions

Contrary to previous advice, since it has been shown that the liver ordinarily clears the blood reaching it completely of the drug—and enzyme inducers obviously cannot increase clearance beyond 100%—there is no requirement to shorten the injection interval. This applies to many on such drugs for epilepsy and even to users of the most powerful enzyme-inducer, rifampicin. This makes it a first-choice option for many long-term users.

Starting routines—timing of the first injection

- In menstruating women, the first injection should ideally be given on day 1, but can be up to day 5 of the cycle; if given later than day 5 (see above) advise 7 days' extra precautions.
- If a woman is on a COC or POP or Cerazette™ up to the day of injection, the injection can normally be given any time, with no added precautions.
- Post-partum (when the woman is not breastfeeding) or after a second-trimester abortion, the first injection should normally be at about day 21, and if later with added precautions for 7 days. If later and still amenorrhoeic, pregnancy risk must be excluded (pp. 166–9). Earlier use has been reported as leading to prolonged heavy bleeding, but is sometimes clinically justified.
- During lactation, if chosen, DMPA is best given at 6 weeks. Lactation is not inhibited at all. The dose to the infant is small, and believed to be entirely harmless beyond 6 weeks.
- After miscarriage or a first-trimester abortion: injection on the day or after expulsion of fetus if a medical procedure was used. If the injection is given beyond the fifth day, advise 7 days' extra precautions.

Overdue injections of DMPA with continuing sexual intercourse

How best to deal with these has caused much debate. In the United Kingdom, conceptions have been reported to the manufacturer as early as the end of the 13th week. However, these are extremely rare and the ongoing anovulatory effect of DMPA in most women is such that, amazingly, WHO now permits the injection to be repeated at 16 weeks plus 1 day! FSRH's view is between these extremes and defines an overdue injection that requires EC with sexual exposure, as 14 weeks plus 1 day. Is *this* soon enough? Might fertility return in some UK women be faster than as reported to WHO? Fortunately, the teratogenic risk if DMPA is given in early pregnancy appears to be very low. The problem is the injection cannot be removed once given, whereas Pills can be stopped if conception occurs.

The box below summarizes my own suggested protocol, modified from FSRH advice in their 2009 Guidance document (URL on page 103):

Protocol for overdue injection - beyond 84 days (12 weeks)

A If has truly abstained since due date (however much now overdue): just give next injection and advise 7 days' added contraception

B If there has been continuing unprotected sexual intercourse (UPSI):

- **From day 85 until day 98 (end of 14th week)**, give the injection plus advise added contraception (condoms) during the next 7 days. Pregnancy testing is rarely helpful.

- **Beyond day 98 (beyond end of 14th week), with earliest UPSI up to 5 days before.** If a pregnancy test today is negative, the next injection can be given *along with hormonal EC* (ellaOne™ preferred as Levonelle™ is ineffective post-ovulation). Added precautions are advised for 7 + 7 = 14 days if ellaOne used (p. 150) and arrange a confirmatory pregnancy test at 21 days after *last* UPSI.

  – Option 2: *a copper IUD* may be fitted for the EC, with choice to transfer to that method, OR if injection also given, have IUD removed after pregnancy test confirms success at 21 days after last UPSI.

- **Beyond day 98 (beyond end of 14th week),** if earliest UPSI was also after day 98 *and* more than 5 days ago (so it is now likely to be more than 5 days beyond a *possible* ovulation), and today's pregnancy test is negative, **EITHER**

  – Reach agreement with the woman that she will (preferably) abstain, otherwise use condoms with greatest care, UNTIL there has been a total of 21 days since the last sexual exposure. If a sensitive (20–25 IU/L) pregnancy test is then negative, the next DMPA dose can be given plus the usual advice for 7 further days of added barrier contraception.

OR

  – If the woman is not prepared to abstain or use condoms for the necessary days to reach 21 since her last sex, a most useful option is *Bridging* with the POP (usually Cerazette) for that time

---

and then proceed as above. The teratogenic risks to a fetus exposed to the POP have been established as very low.

In all the above circumstances, counsel the woman regarding possible failure and the need for a check pregnancy test if there is doubt.

What should NOT happen is the woman who is over 2 weeks late with her injection being told to go away until she has her next period!

Note: DMPA may always be given early, indeed the very earliest in my view could be after the decline in peak blood levels at c. 4 weeks after a previous dose.

ADVANTAGES AND INDICATIONS

DMPA has obvious contraceptive benefits, but it also shares most of the non-contraceptive benefits of the COC described above, including protection against pelvic infection and endometrial cancer. Few metabolic changes have been described.

Main indications
- The woman's desire for a highly effective method that is independent of intercourse and unaffected by enzyme inducers, and
- When other options are contraindicated or disliked.
- A past history of ectopic pregnancy or, like all other progestogen-only methods, of
- Past thrombosis or increased risk—e.g. for effective contraception while waiting for major or leg surgery (Cerazette is another option here).

Non-contraceptive indications
- Endometriosis
- Past symptomatic functional cysts
- Sickle cell anaemia
- Epilepsy, in which it often reduces the frequency of seizures

PROBLEMS AND DISADVANTAGES

Possibly its main one is unique among available contraceptives, that it is impossible to reverse, i.e. to take the injection out again once given, to reverse an effect or side effect of a dose (for at least 3 months, sometimes longer). It is *unfair* not to mention this fact in advance.

Side effects, summarized

- Irregular, sometimes prolonged, bleeding and/or spotting (see box below). ''Structured information' about this, at the start and repeated, has been shown to reduce discontinuation by 12 months. This is probably because perseverance so often leads to amenorrhoea (70% by one year) which can be highly acceptable once it is understood that *'periods don't have any excretory function or health benefits'*
- Amenorrhoea*—a good side effect, but not always so seen
- Delayed return of fertility—something to warn about (see below)
- Weight gain. A Cochrane review found a *mean* weight gain of about 3 kg at 2 years. But some users gain considerably more than this—again, forewarn!
- Some concern regarding reduced bone density—which is probably over-emphasised, but see below
- There are the usual reports of 'minor side effects' such as headache, mood change and loss of libido, yet there is no hard evidence of a causal association with these. With respect to libido, perhaps partly caused by vaginal dryness, lowered estrogen levels may be a factor in individual cases—and clinically finding another effective method has seemed to improve that problem
- Local problems:
  - haematoma very rare, commoner if anticoagulated
  - infection, also rare

*A useful explanation is 'no blood is coming away because there is no blood there TO come away'.

Management of frequent or prolonged bleeding

- First, check that it does not have a non-DMPA-related cause (e.g. *Chlamydia*, but others as relevant from 'D-Checklist', p. 63).
- Advise that it has a better prognosis than with implants, usually being an early problem that is then generally followed by amenorrhoea after 3 to 6 months (70% at 12 months).
- The likelihood of amenorrhoea can be increased by reducing the injection interval (usually to 10 weeks). Otherwise:
- Try additional estrogen, most easily provided as a 30-μg COC. WHO has some evidence of its efficacy. I recommend giving it cyclically (i.e. normally, 21/28) with the rationale that each withdrawal bleed will act like a 'pharmacological curettage', designed to clear out the existing endometrium that is bleeding in an unacceptable way—in the hope that a 'better'

endometrium giving a more acceptable bleeding pattern will be obtained post-treatment. The plan should be explained to the woman, who should also be pre-warned that it may not work.
- Possible treatments are
  - EE 30 µg (as such, or more usually within a Pill formulation such as Microgynon 30™) given daily for 21 days, usually for three cycles. Courses may be repeated, if this helps during the treatment but an acceptable bleeding pattern does not follow, or
  - mefenamic acid 500 mg bd, which in some studies helped to terminate prolonged bleeding episodes, may also be tried.

Bone density and related issues

Most DMPA-users have estradiol (E2) levels similar to the early-to-mid follicular phase but in some women they are decidedly low for women in the fertile years. The question is, does prolonged hypo-estrogenism in some women through use of DMPA lead, by analogy with premature menopause, to added risk of bone density loss or frank osteoporosis; or possibly arterial disease in those already predisposed, such as smokers?

Arterial disease

Studies including WHO (1998) continue to be reassuring with respect to arterial as well as venous circulatory disease and a 1999 cohort study from Thailand found no difference in BP between IUD-users and DMPA-users after 10 years.

Bone mineral density

After more than 30 years of research but still few good studies, there remains uncertainty—not about the variably low follicular-phase estradiol levels that are found in DMPA-users, but about their implications for bone health. We know that:

- Mean bone mineral density (BMD) is lower in DMPA-users than in controls in cross-sectional comparisons, including among women above age 45, but not post-menopausally.
- This finding is unconnected to the bleeding pattern (it may or may not occur in women experiencing either amenorrhoea or irregular bleeding).

- It increases again upon discontinuation (suggestive that this loss is E2 related and a real effect—but also very reassuring for reversibility).
- From limited evidence, the BMD in *adolescent* DMPA-users is lower than controls using implants (or COCs). This has raised the concern that normal peak bone mass might not be fully achieved if DMPA were used during teenage years. On the positive side for teens, however, is the evidence of reversibility (last bullet) and the fact that bone density does not finally peak until age 25. Having a general policy of switching from 3-monthly DMPA to a 3-yearly implant as soon as teens achieve amenorrhoea with the former (which is often in less than a year) will also address this concern (see protocol below).
- Long-term DMPA-using women examined after their *menopause* versus lifetime never-users have not been shown to differ in their bone densities, again suggesting possible recovery of bone mass after stopping.

Based on the above, UKMEC therefore simply states that DMPA is WHO 2 for adolescents and for women over age 45.

How long to use DMPA (UK protocol)?

There is no specified maximum duration, but the CSM circular of November 2004 had one main recommendation, namely 'careful re-evaluation of risks and benefits in all those who wish to continue use for more than 2 years'.

Expanded from this, in the United Kingdom, the following is now advised, clinically:

Protocols for *choice* and *duration* of use of DMPA
First, *if there is known osteopenia or osteoporosis, or strong risk factors for osteoporosis* already exist, DMPA is WHO 4. Examples of the latter:
- Long-term corticosteroid treatment
- Secondary amenorrhoea, due to anorexia nervosa or marathon running
- An untreated malabsorption syndrome (e.g. gluten enteropathy)

However, the category could become WHO 3 if a BMD scan shows no osteopenia, the risk factor has ceased, and the young woman has been obtaining either natural estrogen during normal cycling or EE through the COC.

- *Under age 19,* due to the above concern that it may prevent achievement of peak bone mass, UKMEC classifies DMPA as WHO 2; and the UK advice of November 2004 is similar, namely to use it *first-line* 'but only after other methods have been discussed' and are unsuitable or unacceptable.
- *Above age 45,* DMPA is also WHO 2 (because of the possibility of incipient ovarian failure and also because methods without this concern are available, such as the (old-type) POP, which would be equally effective at this age).

Second, if the method is now chosen:
- DMPA remains a highly effective, safe and 'forgettable' method, usable by almost any woman in the childbearing years.
- Women should be informed that there may be a small loss of BMD, but this is usually recovered after discontinuation.
- In summary, DMPA is now perceived as **primarily a 'Bridging' method (p. 169), very useful for fairly short-term use, after which switching to another long-term method such as an implant would be usual**.
- There should be a regular 'formal' 2-yearly discussion and reassessment of alternatives, but **without blood tests or any imaging. Such (e.g. bone density scanning) would only be appropriate if indicated for that particular woman on specific clinical grounds related to herself.** It is not a routine part of the protocol.
- At one of these 2-yearly discussions, usefully based on the FPA's leaflet *Your Guide to Contraception*, many will therefore choose to switch from DMPA to another long-acting method (e.g. to Nexplanon^TM*, a copper IUD or the IUS) after 2–4–6 years, or above age 45 to a POP. However:
- If instead the woman wishes to use DMPA for longer, it is as always her right to decide to do so, on the 'informed user–chooser' basis, after counselling about the uncertainty.
- It happens that African-Caribbean women have, genetically, higher BMD levels, as do obese women: so the provider may be more comfortable if they wish to use DMPA for a longer duration than others.

*Practical advantages of this particular switch are as follows:
  – The implant can be 'sold' as being essentially the same as their existing DMPA but with an injection every 3 years rather than every 3 months.
  – There is a strong clinical impression that if the DMPA-user has amenorrhoea, this reduces the risk of unacceptable bleeding when the implant is inserted—at least for the first year.
  – The implant can be inserted at a time that suits everyone rather than having to be in the first 5 days of the cycle (see p. 110).

Remember, when all is said and done, that the safety issue of osteoporosis with DMPA is much less important than the potentially lethal rare complications of EE within CHCs.

Are there not similar bone density concerns with long-term Nexplanon™?

There are not. The data are reassuring so far: in a non-randomized comparative study described below, after 2 years, estradiol levels and bone densities remained similar among Nexplanon-users to those among copper IUD–users. By analogy, since Cerazette is a bit like 'oral Implanon™', there are no worries yet on this account with Cerazette either—nor with the IUS (below), whose amenorrhoeic action is anyway primarily at the end-organ level (the endometrium).

CONTRAINDICATIONS

These are similar to the POP (JG's opinion) but affected by the higher dose and lack of immediate reversibility of DMPA.

Absolute contraindications for DMPA (WHO 4)

- Current *osteopenia or osteoporosis* on scan or severe risk factor(s) for osteoporosis as above, including chronic corticosteroid treatment (>5 mg prednisolone/day)
- Any serious adverse effect of COCs not certainly related solely to the estrogen content (e.g. *liver adenoma or cancer*—although UKMEC classifies these as WHO 3)
- *Recent breast cancer* not yet clearly in remission (see below)
- History of *acute porphyria* (progestogens as well as estrogens are believed capable of precipitating these, 1% of attacks are fatal and the injection is not 'removable')
- *Hypersensitivity* to any component
- Actual or possible *pregnancy*

WHO 3 conditions for DMPA

- Factors suggesting *high risk of osteoporosis* but normal or minimally reduced BMD on bone scan
- Current ischaemic heart disease, *severe arterial diseases* including stroke (because of the above evidence about low

---

estrogen levels coupled with reports of lowered HDL cholesterol) and current VTE
- *Diabetes with any evidence of tissue damage or of >20 years duration*
- *Familial hyperlipidaemias* (other progestogen-only methods such as the POP or Cerazette are preferred for all the above)
- *Breast cancer, in complete remission* (after 5 years according to UKMEC). However, a POP or LNG-IUS would be preferable (lower dose, more reversible)
- *Severe liver disease* (acute viral hepatitis, decompensated cirrhosis)
- Undiagnosed *genital tract bleeding* until cause established

WHO 2 conditions for DMPA

- Under 18 or over 45 years of age are WHO 2 with respect to the bones (see above)
- History of VTE, any predisposition to VTE
- Obesity, although further weight gain is *not* inevitable (see below)
- Hypertension, controlled on treatment
- Hyperlipidaemias other than familial type (take advice)
- Strong *family history of breast cancer*—UKMEC says WHO 1 for this.
- *Known BRCA mutation* present
- Cervical cancer or CIN awaiting treatment
- Active liver disease: compensated cirrhosis, with moderately abnormal liver function
- Gallbladder disease
- Cholestasis history, CHC related
- Porphyrias other than the acute intermittent variety
- Bleeding tendency. This is WHO 2 because of deep haematoma risk, minimized by extra care when injections are given. With the INR in the normal range (2–3) warfarin treatment is similarly only WHO 2—and does not contraindicate (WHO 1) Nexplanon, which is inserted so superficially
- Breastfeeding <6 weeks post-partum
- Past severe endogenous depression (UKMEC says WHO 1)
- Undiagnosed genital tract bleeding
- Planning a pregnancy in the near future
- Unwillingness to cope with prospect of irregularity or absence of periods
  – sometimes connected with cultural/religious taboos

COUNSELLING

Aside from taking account of the WHO eligibility factors above, there are four main practical points that *must* be made to prospective users:

- *The effects, whether wanted (contraceptive) or unwanted, are not reversible for the duration of the injection:* this fact is unique among current contraceptives.
- Weight gain, though no study has proved causation by any other hormonal contraceptives, is uniquely for real with DMPA. It is believed to be due to increased appetite, so it is useful (and can really work) to advise a pre-emptive plan to start taking extra exercise as well as watching diet. It may help some women's decision-making that those who are not already overweight put on significantly less than those who are.
- Irregular, sometimes prolonged, bleeding may be a problem, but the outlook is good (see above).
- After the last dose, conception is commonly delayed with a median delay of 9 months since the last injection, which is of course only around 6 months after cessation of the method. However, in some individuals it could be well over 1 year, and all should be warned of that possibility. A comparative study in Thailand showed that almost 95% of previously fertile users had conceived by 28 months after their last injection. So there is no evidence of permanent infertility caused by the drug. With respect to continuing post-DMPA amenorrhoea:
  - If conception **is not** wanted, alternative contraception must begin from about 13 weeks since the last injection.
  - If conception **is** wanted, spontaneous ovulation can be anticipated in most cases: if not, refer for investigation ± treatment at about 12 months after the last injection.

FOLLOW-UP

Aside from ensuring the injections take place at the correct intervals, follow-up is primarily advisory and supportive:

- Prolonged or too frequent bleeding is managed as already described.
- BP is normally checked initially, but there is absolutely no need for it to be taken before each dose, as studies fail to show any hypertensive effect. An annual check is reasonable as well-woman care. Roll on the option of self-administration (Uniject p. 92)!

For more on injectables including most of the important references, visit
www.fsrh.org/pdfs/CEUGuidanceProgestogenOnlyInjectables09.pdf
- last updated 2009.

The commonest implants worldwide contain a progestogen in a slow-release carrier, made either of dimethylsiloxane, as in Jadelle™ or Sino-implant (11)™ (not available in the United Kingdom) with two implants, or ethylene vinyl acetate (EVA), as in Nexplanon™ otherwise known in some locations as Implanon NXT, a single rod (Fig. 13).

They are excellent examples of long-acting reversible contraceptives (LARCs), with the ideal 'forgettable' default state, yet rapid reversibility.

MECHANISM OF ACTION, ADMINISTRATION AND EFFECTIVENESS

Nexplanon, formerly known as Implanon, works primarily by ovulation inhibition, supplemented mainly by the usual sperm-blocking mucus effect. It is a single 40-mm rod, just 2 mm in diameter, containing 68 mg of etonogestrel—the chief active metabolite of desogestrel—and so has much in common with Cerazette™. This is dispersed in an EVA matrix and covered by a 0.06-mm rate-limiting EVA membrane. The rod now also contains barium sulphate, so it can be imaged by X ray but it remains bio-equivalent to Implanon, with the same release rate and 3-year licensed duration of action.

Useful Faculty Guidance on implants can be accessed at www.fsrh.org/pdfs/CEUStatementNexplanon1110.pdf and www.fsrh.org/pdfs/CEUGuidanceProgestogenOnlyImplantsApril08.pdf

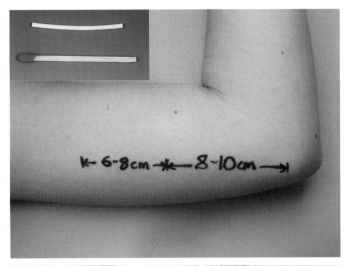

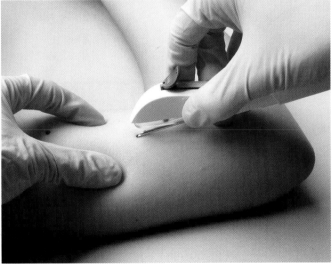

Figure 13

Nexplanon^TM, *showing positioning and marking up of the arm and subsequent use of new inserter system. Source: Courtesy of Dr Anne MacGregor.*

Nexplanon—the main points summarized

- Nexplanon is inserted subdermally but very superficially under the skin over the biceps, medially in the upper arm, under local anaesthesia, from a dedicated sterile pre-loaded applicator by a simple one-handed injection-and-withdrawal technique. Note the positioning of the recipient's arm (Fig. 13). The provider should be seated so as to see the progress of the needle, following the instructions provided with the product.

- Current teaching, following the revised SPC, is to insert away from and usually anterior to the groove between the triceps and biceps, hence superficial to the biceps muscle and well away from the neurovascular bundle.

- Although this implant is much easier than Norplant was both to insert or to remove, specific ('model arm' plus live) training is essential and cannot be obtained from any book. In the United Kingdom, the best training is obtainable through the FSRH to obtain their Letter of Competence (LoC) in sub-dermal implants (SDIs). Details of the required e-learning and practical training may be found at www.fsrh.org/pdfs/FormX.pdf.

- After an initial phase of several weeks giving higher blood levels, Nexplanon delivers almost constant low daily levels of the hormone, for a recommended duration of use of 3 years.

- In the pre-marketing trials, Nexplanon had the unique distinction of a zero failure rate. The 'perfect use' failure rate is now estimated as about 5 in 10,000 insertions (Table 1), so since 'user failures' are improbable it shares the status with the LNG implants of *most effective reversible contraceptives ever devised*.

- Most of the 'failures' that have been reported either had had the insertion during a conception cycle or were failures to insert at all.

- *Effect of body mass?* In the international studies, serum levels tended to be lower in overweight women, but, in the post-marketing study, failures attributed to high body mass have not been reported. It is unclear whether this is because providers have been offering other methods to grossly overweight women or replacing implants early as advised by the SPC—or a function of the 'margin of safety' of this incredibly effective method.

- However, clinically, it is clear this finding should not deter providers from offering Nexplanon to overweight women as a medically safer option than any CHC (especially Evra™), with respect to VTE risk (see below).

- Reversibility is normally simple by removal of the implant, with almost immediate effect.

MAINTAINING EFFECTIVENESS
The main causes of failure

All are rare, but include

- insertion during a conception cycle—discussed below (p. 110);
- failures to insert at all—should now be vanishingly rare, given the new inserter technology plus the advice that both provider and user *always* palpate the Nexplanon in situ just after insertion;
- enzyme-inducing drugs.

What about body weight?

Is this relevant? See Box above (7th bullet). The SPC states:

> The contraceptive effect of Nexplanon is related to the plasma levels of etonogestrel, which are inversely related to body weight, and decrease with time after insertion ... It cannot be excluded that the contraceptive effect in these women during the third year of use may be lower than for women of normal weight. HCPs [healthcare providers] may therefore consider earlier replacement of the implant in heavier women.

The word 'consider' there is unclear for providers: my own practice would be *only* to discuss earlier replacement with a young fertile woman with weight well over 100 kg, if she also began to cycle regularly in the third year (suggesting reliance only on the mucus effect).

Enzyme-inducer drug treatment

The SPC states that hepatic enzyme inducers may lower the blood levels of etonogestrel, but there have been no specific interaction studies. Therefore, women on *short-term treatment* with any of these drugs are advised to use a barrier method in addition and (because reversal of enzyme induction always takes time) for 28 days thereafter. *During long-term enzyme-inducer drug* treatment, MSD recommends transfer to an unaffected method and removal of the Nexplanon. This seems a bit wasteful, may be resisted by satisfied users—and those in monogamous relationships may reject the long-term use of barriers. A possible approach, clearly unlicensed (see pp. 173–175) and without FSRH endorsement, would be (in my view) to attempt to compensate by either adding a daily Cerazette even more controversially, a second Nexplanon—there are no studies. However, since enzyme-inducer drug users do so well with DMPA or the IUD or IUS, these are definitely the preferred choices for long-term users.

ADVANTAGES AND INDICATIONS

The main indication is the woman's desire for a highly effective yet at all times rapidly reversible method, without the finality of sterilization, which is independent of intercourse: especially when other options are contraindicated or disliked.

- Above all, it provides efficacy and convenience: if the bleeding pattern suits, it is a 'forgettable' contraceptive.
- Long duration of action with one treatment (3 years)—a 'selling-point when switching from DMPA—and high continuation rates.
- There is no initial peak dose given orally to the liver.
- Blood levels are low and fairly steady, rather than fluctuating (as with the POP) or initially too high (as with injectables); this, with the previous point, means metabolic changes are few and believed to be negligible.
- Nexplanon is estrogen-free, and therefore definitely usable if there is a history of VTE (WHO 2).
- Median systolic and diastolic BP were unchanged in trials for up to 4 years.
- Being an anovulant, special indications include past ectopic pregnancy.
- The effects are rapidly reversible, an advantage over DMPA, which is worth emphasizing. After removal, serum etonogestrel levels are undetectable after 4 days, so return of fertility must be assumed to be almost immediate.

CONTRAINDICATIONS

Contraindications are very similar to Cerazette since Nexplanon is an anovulant, yet, unlike DMPA, immediately reversible—and they contain essentially the same progestogen.

Absolute contraindications (WHO 4) for Nexplanon

- Any serious adverse effect of COCs not certainly related solely to the estrogen (e.g. liver adenoma or cancer: UKMEC is more permissive, WHO 3)
- Recent breast cancer not yet clearly in remission (see below)
- Known or suspected pregnancy
- Hypersensitivity to any component

WHO 3 conditions for Nexplanon

- Current ischaemic heart disease, *severe arterial diseases* including stroke
- Sex-steroid-dependent cancer, including *breast cancer*, when in complete remission (UKMEC states WHO 4 until 5 years, then WHO 3). Agreement of the relevant hospital consultant should be obtained and the woman's autonomy respected: record that she understands it is unknown whether progestogen might alter the recurrence risk (either way)
- *Severe liver disease* (acute viral hepatitis, decompensated cirrhosis)
- *Acute porphyria*, if there is a history of actual attack triggered by sex hormones (my view, since progestogens as well as estrogens are believed capable of precipitating these attacks and 1% are fatal). Otherwise, the history of acute porphyria is WHO 2
- Undiagnosed *genital tract bleeding* until cause established
- *Enzyme-inducer drugs*. Although very exceptionally, in my view, an added Cerazette daily might be taken, off licence (pp. 173–175), another method such as an injectable, IUD or IUS would be preferable

WHO 2 conditions for Nexplanon

- *Current VTE* (UKMEC says WHO 3), *past VTE* or marked risk factors/*predispositions to VTE*
- *Risk factors for arterial disease* or current high risk including diabetes with arteriopathy; hypertension: more than one risk factor can be present, in contrast to COCs
- Strong *family history of breast cancer*—UKMEC says WHO 1 for this
- *Known BRCA mutation* present
- *Current liver disorder*—even if there is persistent biochemical change—including compensated cirrhosis, history of CHC-related cholestasis
- *Gall bladder disease*

- Most other *chronic severe systemic diseases* including inflammatory bowel disease (but WHO 3 if there is significant malabsorption of sex steroids)
- Past *symptomatic (painful) functional ovarian cysts*. But persistent cysts/follicles that are commonly detected on routine ultrasonography can be disregarded if they caused no symptoms
- Unwillingness to cope with prospect of irregularity or absence of periods
  - sometimes connected with cultural/religious taboos

TIMING OF NEXPLANON™ INSERTION

- **In the woman's natural cycle**, day 1–5 is usual timing; if any day later than day 5 (provided no sexual exposure up to that day), recommend additional contraception for 7 days.
- If a woman is on COC or POP/Cerazette or DMPA, the implant can normally be inserted at any time, overlapping with the other method, with no added precautions.

Clinical implications

Insertions only during the above tiny natural-cycle window are a logistic nightmare! There is also pressure on providers, when women arrive later in the cycle without 'believable abstinence' or full security about condom use, to insert anyway.

So a useful practical tip is to actively recommend *as the normal routine*, at counselling, the use or re-use of an anovulant method (i.e. one of those in the second bullet point above), to continue until the Nexplanon insertion.

An extension of this concept is to *recommend to Nexplanon requesters that they defer the insertion until they have achieved amenorrhoea through DMPA injections, as many or as few as they need to have stopped all bleeding for (say) 60 days—and insert only after that.* This often occurs after two to four injections (p. 96) and clinical experience suggests (though we badly need the results of a planned clinical trial to prove the point) that this will reduce the risk of unacceptable bleeding in the weeks following the insertion.

Timing in non-cycling states

- Following delivery (not breastfeeding) or second-trimester abortion, insertion on about day 21 is recommended, or if later with additional contraception for 7 days. If later and still amenorrhoeic, pregnancy risk should be excluded, often by 'Bridging' first with a POP for 3 weeks followed by a negative pregnancy test (p. 169).
- If breastfeeding, insert ideally on day 21 with no need for added contraception for 7 days. Reassurance can be given that the implant can safely be used in lactation—the infant receiving c. 0.2% of estimated maternal dose.
- Following first-trimester abortion, immediate insertion is best
  – on the day of surgically induced abortion or the second part of a medical abortion, or
  – up to 5 days later
  – if >5 days later, an added method such as condoms is recommended for 7 days.
- To follow any other effective contraceptive (CHC, POP, DMPA, IUD, IUS), it is often best to overlap the methods by at least 7 days: so there is no loss of protection between methods and no need to discuss supplementary condom use.
- To replace a previous Nexplanon after 3 years, the new one may be inserted through the same removal incision (see p. 114), with additional local anaesthetic and ensuring that the needle is inserted to its full length.

COUNSELLING AND ONGOING SUPERVISION

Explain always the likely changes to the bleeding pattern and the possibility of 'hormonal' side effects (see below). This discussion should as always be backed by a good leaflet, such as the FPA one, and well documented.

No treatment-specific follow-up is necessary (including no need for BP checks). The SPC recommends the option of one follow-up visit at 3 months. More important is an explicit 'open-house' policy, so the woman knows she can return at any time to discuss possible side effects and their treatment (see below), without any provider pressure to persevere if the woman really wants the implant removed (the service standard for the maximum wait for removal should be no more than 2 weeks).

Bleeding problems

- Experience shows that around 50% to 60% of women have a bleeding pattern that, though not regular, is acceptably light and infrequent, so most of these continue with the method. Of the remainder:
- About 20% develop amenorrhoea by 1 year and with forewarning and reassurance (p. 96) most will persevere.
- About 20% have frequent or prolonged bleeding and spotting. Whatever is experienced in the first 3 months is broadly predictive of future bleeding patterns.

Clinical management of unacceptable bleeding

With reassurance, most women are happy to accept one of the patterns in the first two groups above. For the third group, perseverance beyond 3 months is rewarded less often than with DMPA (or the IUS). *After eliminating unrelated causes for the bleeding* (p. 63), which as usual is crucial, e.g. *Chlamydia* infection:

- The best short-term treatment is cyclical estrogen therapy to produce those 'pharmacological curettages' (i.e. withdrawal bleeds), on a similar basis to the above regimen for DMPA (pp. 96–97). This may most easily be provided by three cycles of Mercilon or more often Marvelon (with 30 μg of EE), after which the bleeding may (or sometimes may not!) become acceptable. This plan should be explained in advance to the woman, who should also understand that it is not certain to work. Courses may be repeated if an acceptable bleeding pattern does not follow. Or,
- If the above approach fails or the woman has a WHO 4 contra-indication to EE, an alternative based on data extrapolated from studies with LNG implants is to try a short course of mefenamic acid 500 mg bd.
- Some clinicians report that empirically giving added Cerazette tablet daily has 'worked' enough times to be worth a try.

We badly need good RCTs to establish the value or otherwise of the above regimens. Personally, I favour the policy above, of attempting to *pre-empt* annoying bleeding problems *by creating amenorrhoea first,* using DMPA—though whether this approach works long term (rather than just for the first c. 12–18 months) also needs confirmation.

> **Minor side effects**
>
> Reported in frequency order, minor side effects were
> - Acne (but this also sometimes improved!)
> - Headache
> - Abdominal pain
> - Breast pain
> - 'Dizziness'
> - Mood changes (depression, emotional lability)
> - Libido decrease
> - Hair loss

There is no scientific proof of a causal link between the implant and any of the symptoms in the box above—including the often-alleged problems of weight gain, mood change and loss of libido. However, users should always be 'met where they are'—and if they are convinced that their symptom is related to the implant, and unacceptable, they need to be actively helped to find an alternative acceptable method.

> **Local adverse effects** may also occur, namely:
> - infection of the site
> - expulsion
> - migration and difficult removal
> - scarring (very rare)

Bone mineral density

Since Nexplanon suppresses ovulation and does not supply any estrogen, the same questions as with DMPA arise over possible hypo-estrogenism. However, in a non-randomized comparative study, no estradiol or bone density differences in the means, ranges or standard errors were detected between 44 users of Nexplanon and 29 users of copper IUDs over 2 years, which is reassuring, pending more data.

It appears that, as for Cerazette and the other POPs, the suppression of FSH levels with Nexplanon is less complete, allowing generally higher follicular estrogen levels than there are in (some) users of DMPA.

Reversibility and removal problems

Reversal is normally simple, with almost immediate effect. Under local anaesthesia, steady digital pressure on the proximal end of the Nexplanon after a 2-mm incision over the distal end leads to delivery of that end of the rod, removal being completed by grasping it with mosquito forceps. As for insertion, removal training is crucial, using the 'model arm' and also live under supervision.

Removal problems can be minimized by good training, in both the insertion and removal techniques. Difficult removals correlate with initially too-deep insertion. Beware particularly of the thin or very muscular woman with very little subcutaneous tissue. Insertion can easily permit a segment of the rod to enter an arm muscle, with deep migration following.

A plain X ray will display a 'lost' Nexplanon, but its removal may need to be under ultrasound control. The manufacturer at www.msd-uk.com should be contacted for advice and help in all such cases.

Intrauterine contraception

Intrauterine contraceptives are currently of two distinct types:

- Copper intrauterine devices (IUDs), in which the copper ion (the actual contraceptive) is released from a band or wire on a plastic carrier.
- The levonorgestrel-releasing intrauterine system, which releases that progestogen—this will be abbreviated below as either LNG-IUS or just IUS.

The latest Faculty Guidance on intrauterine contraception can be accessed at www.fsrh.org/pdfs/CEUGuidanceIntrauterineContraceptionNov07.pdf— along with 133 references that give support to this chapter.

COPPER-BEARING DEVICES

'It is time to forgive the intrauterine device!'

This headline to an article says it all. Actually, there are over 150 million users worldwide, but the lion's share is in just one country—China. It seems improbable that the difference between less than 1% of sexually active users in United States or 5% in the United Kingdom but 20% in France is explicable by some important difference between the French, the British and the US uterus. Do the Chinese and the French have something to teach the rest of the world?

In many countries, women in their late 30s have not been requesting IUDs because they were told by their mothers to avoid that method. This is unfortunate, because in reality a woman in her later reproductive years with, say, two or three children, is the ideal user. The devices have changed over the years but more importantly she has too—a parous cervical canal makes insertion easier and commonly she also has less exposure to STIs than in her youth.

Some doctors are complying too readily with requests for male or female sterilization that originate partly from 'medical myths' about the intrauterine alternative. Leaving aside the significant advance represented by the LNG-IUS, too few women know that the latest **banded copper IUDs** (Fig. 14) are, in practice, comparable to reversible sterilization.

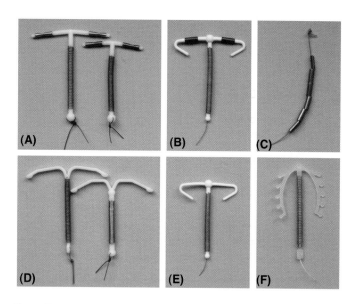

Figure 14

Copper IUDs. (A) TT 380 Slimline (Durbin) and Mini TT 380 Slimline (Durbin) with short stem. T-Safe Cu 380A QL (Quick Load) (Williams). T-Safe 380A Capped (Williams). (B) Flexi-T+380 (Durbin). (C) GyneFix (Williams). (D) UT 380 Standard (Durbin) and UT 380 Short (Durbin) with short stem. Nova T380 (Bayer). Neo-Safe T380 (Williams). (E) Flexi-T 300 (Durbin) Cu-Safe T300 (Williams). (F) Multiload Cu375 (MSD) Load 375 (Durbin). Source: Courtesy of Dr Anne MacGregor.

> **Advantages of copper IUDs and of the IUS—a long list!**
> - *Safe*: mortality 1:500,000
> - *Effective*:
>   - Immediately (slower for the IUS)
>   - Post-coitally (this is not true of the LNG-IUS)
>   - Highly, like sterilization if one of the many clones of the T-Safe Cu 380A is used (see below)
> - *No link with coitus*
> - *No tablets* to remember
> - *Continuation rates are high* and permitted duration of use can exceed 10 years
> - *Reversible*—and there is evidence that this is true even when they have been removed for one of the recognized complications
> - A systematic review (2002) found that copper IUDs *may reduce the risk of endometrial cancer*. This needs confirmation, along with the very possible similar effect of the LNG-IUS (which does undoubtedly protect the endometrium against the otherwise increased rate of this cancer in HRT-users)

Mechanism of action

- Appropriate studies indicate that copper IUDs operate primarily by preventing fertilization, the copper ion being toxic to sperm.
- Their effectiveness when put in post-coitally shows that they act additionally to block implantation. However, when IUDs are in situ long term, this is a secondary or backup mechanism.

> **Clinical implication**
> - As in any given cycle, this type of IUD might be working through the block of implantation, there is a small risk of 'iatrogenic' conception if a device is removed after mid-cycle, even if abstinence follows.
> - Ideally, therefore, women should either use another method additionally from 7 days before planned device removal, or if this has not been the case, postpone removal until the next menses.
> - If a device must be removed earlier, hormonal post-coital contraception may be indicated.

Choice of devices and effectiveness

In the United Kingdom, *the 'gold standard' among IUDs for a parous woman without menstrual problems* (if these are present, a LNG-IUS would be preferable) is *a banded copper IUD* (Fig. 14).

The nomenclature of the devices available is a nightmare! (Fig. 14): they include the generic T-Safe Cu 380A with new variants with their copper bands sunk into the arms of the plastic frame, which are branded as TT 380 'Slimline' or T-Safe Cu 380A QL 'Quick Load' (these are available, respectively, from Durbin and FP Sales—see British National Formulary, BNF).

In Sivin's Population Council randomized controlled trial, this banded IUD type had statistically similar efficacy to the LNG-IUS. The cumulative failure rate of the CuT 380Ag to 10 years was only 1.4 per 100 women (compare a mean rate of 1.8 per 100 women at 10 years after female sterilization in the American CREST study from 1996). There were no failures at all after year 5!

The banded copper device is therefore like 'reversible sterilization'— at least as performed in the United States prior to 1996. But a WHO trial (referenced in FSRH Guidance, 2007) suggests the IUS may be even more effective and the US data of Table 1 show the same.

Important influence of age on effectiveness

Copper IUDs are much more effective in the older woman— largely because of declining fertility. Over the age of 30, there is also a reduction in rates of expulsion and of PID—the latter is believed not to be the result of the older uterus resisting infection but rather because the older woman is generally less exposed to risk of infection (whether through her own lifestyle or that of her partner).

Advantages of one of the banded IUDs

The efficacy of the T-Safe Cu 380A in one randomized controlled trial was greater than that of the all-wire Nova T380. It is licensed for 10 years and the data support effectiveness until 12 years (even when fitted below age 40, see below). But the main advantage lies in the infrequency of re-insertions. Research in the past 50 years has so clearly shown the truth of both of the following slogans:

IUD Slogan 1
Insertion can be a factor in the causation of almost every category of IUD problems.

IUD Slogan 2
Most device-related problems become less common with increasing duration of use ….

Therefore, why would one ever use a 5-year device when a 10-year one will fit? Fewer insertions plus expected benefit from long-term use adds up to 'banded is best!'

What if the woman is nulliparous?

Note that nulliparity per se is not WHO 4 for this method, despite the clinical practice of many doctors suggesting this! Indeed above age 20, UKMEC classifies it as WHO 1/UKMEC 1. The T-Safe Cu 380A and its clones, the 'Slimline' and 'Quick Load', are not necessarily too large, but the first choice now for nulli-parae is the Mini TT 380 Slimline (Durbin), with reduced dimensions but exactly the same amount of copper. Therefore, it must be usable for the same 10-year minimum duration as the larger variant, and approval for this is being sought (2012). Its insertion tube is unfortunately no thinner, yet it usually passes readily through the nulliparous cervix, possibly after minimal dilatation.

Otherwise, for a comfortable and satisfactory fitting, one of the small wire-bearing IUDs may be better (see the options below), with the caveat of possibly reduced efficacy and certainly reduced duration of use.

When to use other IUDs (e.g. Nova T380 and its clones) (Fig. 14)

For emergency contraception (EC)
The Nova T380/Neo-safe T 380/UT 380 Standard or the shorter UT 380 Short[TM] might be appropriate for a nulliparous woman using it for EC and planning (see p. 146) to have the device removed later, once

---

established on a new method (such as say DMPA). Another good EC option for such nulliparae is the Flexi-T 300/Cu-Safe T300, which is exceptionally small and has an easy push-in fitting technique with no separate plunger. But it has been reported to have a fairly high expulsion rate.

Difficult fittings

- For long-term use, the **Nova T380** and the **UT 380 Short** (Nova T style but on a shorter stem, from Durbin) should usually be reserved for when the T-Safe Cu 380A or equivalent cannot be fitted, for some reason. The reason could be an unusually tight cervix or acute flexion of the uterus—rare in parous women but not uncommon in nulliparae.

- There is now also available the **Flexi-T + 380,** on a slightly larger frame and with the advantage of bands on its sidearms but otherwise identical in shape. We need more data on this—sought but not so far forthcoming! It might be very effective and usable for longer than its 5-year licensed life, be as easily inserted as the Flexi-T 300, and have an acceptable expulsion rate. If all that were true, in difficult cases, being copper-banded, it might come to rival the T-Safe Cu 380A and its clones, above. At present, we lack the data to be sure.

- The **Multiload IUDs**, even the 375 thicker wire versions, were— in most of the randomized controlled trials—generally significantly less effective than the T-Safe Cu 380A, with no firm evidence of the reputed better expulsion rate.

When to use the banded but frameless GyneFix? (Fig. 14)

This unique frameless device features a knot that is embedded by its special inserter system in the fundal myometrium. Below the knot, its polypropylene thread bears six copper bands and locates them within the uterine cavity. Being frameless, it is less likely to cause uterine pain, and when correctly inserted it appears to rival the efficacy of the T-Safe Cu 380A. Unfortunately, in routine UK practice it was found to have a high (rather than the expected low) expulsion rate—and all users should be forewarned about the observed risk of unrecognized expulsion. Being able to feel the threads is particularly important with GyneFix.

IF it is available (by referral to someone trained in the specific insertion skills required), indications for GyneFix include:
- Distorted cavity on ultrasound scan (if IUD useable at all)
- A small uterine cavity sounding <6 cm (rival and probably more available options if the uterus sounds to over 5 cm are the **Flexi-T 300/Cu-Safe T300 and the UT 380 Short**). *Beware: short cavities are rare, may only have sounded the cervix . . .*
- Previous history of expulsion or removal of a framed device that was accompanied by excessive cramping, within hours or days of insertion

Fortunately, since the names of copper IUDs are so confusing, from now onwards all mentions of either 'IUD' or 'copper IUD' will refer, unless otherwise stated, only to the banded **T-Safe Cu 380A** or one of its easy-loading variants.

Main problems and disadvantages of copper IUDs

The main medical problems are listed in the following box and dealt with in more detail thereafter. This is actually a remarkably short list as compared with the hormonal methods.

Possible problems with copper IUDs
1. Intrauterine pregnancy—hence its risks, including miscarriage
2. Extrauterine pregnancy—as this is prevented less well than intrauterine (although the absolute risk is definitely reduced in population terms)
3. Expulsion—giving again the risks of pregnancy/miscarriage
4. Perforation, with
   - risks to bowel/bladder and again
   - risks of pregnancy
5. Pelvic infection—as with (2), the IUD is not causative but it is not protective either
6. Malpositioning—which predisposes to (1), (3) and (7)
7. Pain
8. Bleeding which can be
   - increased amount
   - increased duration

Note, clinically from above that:

This means that all of the first six problems need to be excluded as diagnoses before pain and bleeding are ascribed simply to being side effects of this method.

In situ conception

If the woman wishes to go on to full-term pregnancy, after a pelvic ultrasound scan, the device should normally be removed—in the first trimester. This is counter-intuitive, because one would think that this would increase the miscarriage rate. The truth is the reverse: for example, with in situ failures of the Copper T 200 device, the normal rate of spontaneous abortion was 55%, dropping to 20% if the device was removed. The woman should of course be warned that an increased risk of miscarriage still remains.

Other clinical points:
- If the woman is going to have a termination of her pregnancy, her IUD (or IUS) can be removed at the planned surgery; however, it is safest to remove it before any medical abortion.
- If the threads are already missing when she is seen and other causes are excluded, aided by an ultrasound scan (see below): the pregnancy is at increased risk of
  – second-trimester abortion (which could be infected)
  – antepartum haemorrhage
  – premature labour.
- If the woman goes on to full term, it is essential to identify clearly the device in the products of conception. If it is not found, a postpartum X ray should be arranged in case the device is embedded or malpositioned or has perforated. There have been medicolegal cases when this was not done, because of an undiagnosed perforation, or because of unnecessary tests and treatments for 'infertility' when trying for a later wanted pregnancy, caused by a much earlier malpositioned IUD with no visible threads remaining in situ, ever since the original delivery.

There is no evidence of associated **teratogenicity** with conception during or immediately after use of copper devices.

IUDs with 'lost threads'

This symptom of 'lost threads' links together points (1), (3) and (4) in the box on p. 121. There are at least six causes of this condition—three with and three without pregnancy. An intra-abdominal IUD is just as useless at stopping pregnancy as one that has been totally expelled. More commonly, the woman is already pregnant and the threads have been drawn up or the device has altered its position in situ.

IUD Slogan 4
The woman with 'lost threads' is already pregnant until proven otherwise—moreover, even if not yet pregnant, she is likely to be unprotected and at risk of becoming pregnant.

'Lost threads'—six possible causes

Pregnant	Not pregnant
Unrecognized expulsion + pregnancy	Unrecognized expulsion + not yet pregnant
Perforation + pregnancy	Perforation + not yet pregnant
Device in situ + pregnancy	Device in situ + malpositioned or threads short (in uterus, if not found in cervical canal)

Diagnosis and management may involve some or all of the examinations and techniques shown in Figure 15. In this flow diagram, the later stages should follow referral to a specialist.

More about perforation

This has a general estimated risk for all IUDs of about 1 (or no more than 2) per 1000 insertions, but the exact rate (as for expulsion) depends much less on the IUD design than on the skill of the clinician. Perforated devices should now almost always be removable at laparoscopy.

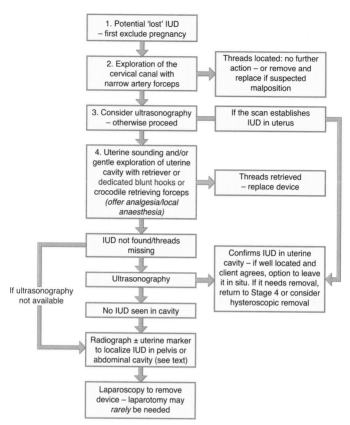

Figure 15
Management of 'lost' IUD threads.

Pelvic inflammatory disease and IUDs—what is the truth?

This is the great fear we all have about IUDs. Just as the Pill has been blamed for problems that we now know were due to smoking, copper IUDs have been blamed for infections that were really acquired sexually (see the Chinese evidence, below).

Much of the anxiety derived from the Dalkon Shield disaster—but this was a unique device with a polyfilamentous thread, facilitating the transfer by capillary action of potential pathogens from the lower to the upper genital tract. Modern copper devices have a monofilamentous thread. They do not themselves cause infection.

However, they provide no protection against PID (in contrast to the LNG-IUS: which may protect slightly, see pp. 133–4), and there is some suspicion that the infections that occur may perhaps be more severe as a result of the foreign-body effect.

In a classic WHO study, Farley et al. (Lancet 1992; 339:785–788) reported on a database from a number of WHO randomized controlled trials including approximately 23,000 insertions of copper IUDs or the LNG-IUS, worldwide. In every country but one, the same pattern emerged (Fig. 16):

- There was an IUD-associated increased risk of infection for 20 days after the insertion.
- However, the weekly infection rate 3 weeks after insertion went back to the same weekly rate as existed before insertion, i.e. the norm for that particular society.

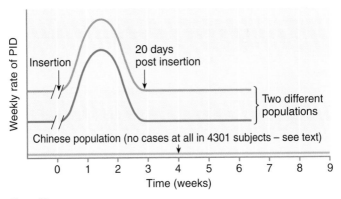

Figure 16
WHO study of 22,908 IUD insertions (4301 in China) in Europe, Africa, Asia and the Americas. Note that the weekly rate of pelvic inflammatory disease (PID) returns to the pre-insertion background rate for the population studied.

In China, the one exception, there were no infections diagnosed at all in spite of 4301 insertions.

Interpretation
These findings are interpreted as follows:

- The post-insertion 'hump' of infections cannot be the result of a bad insertion technique, restricted to doctors outside China.
- It is much more likely that, although the doctors in all the centres were searching for truly monogamous STI-free couples, they were only successful in this search in China (during the 1980s, when it is well recognized that China was practically an STI-free zone—China is no longer unique in this respect today).
- In the other countries, PID-causing organisms (especially *Chlamydia trachomatis*) are presumed to have been present—no cervical pre-screening being available at that time—in a proportion of the women. The process of insertion would interfere with natural defensive mechanisms (as has been confirmed when there is instrumentation in other contexts, such as therapeutic abortion).
- This would enable organisms to spread from the lower genital tract, where they had previously resided asymptomatically, into the upper genital tract, so causing the PID.

In summary, therefore:

IUD/IUS Slogan 5
The devices, intrinsically, cannot be the cause of the PID that occurs in IUD/IUS-users.
[Otherwise, how improbable it is that there would have been 4301 Chinese users in the 1980s research and not a single reported attack!]

- The greatest infection risk is in the first 20 days, most probably caused by pre-existing carriage of STIs.
- Risk thereafter, as with pre-insertion, relates to the background risk of STIs (high in Africa, but so low in mainland China in the 1980s that it seems to have been absent in the study population).

Therefore, the evidence-based policy should be that:

- Elective IUD insertions and re-insertions should always occur through a 'Chinese cervix', i.e. one that has been established to be pathogen-free, so hopefully eliminating the post-insertion infections shown in Figure 16.

Clinical implications for IUD insertion arrangements

- Prospective IUD-users should always be verbally screened, meaning a good sexual history (p. 7). They need to know that they will need to use condoms too if the method is judged WHO 3 because of situational high STI risk—or even abandon this choice and use another method altogether (WHO 4).
- Also—and this is the thorny one we all tend to leave out—'Do you ever wonder if your partner has or is likely to have another sexual relationship?' (Reworded as appropriate, and always with the utmost tact.)
- In populations with high prevalence of *C. trachomatis* (say >5% incidence, and usually for those under 25), this verbal screen should be backed by DNA-based *Chlamydia* pre-screening. This is as important for re-insertions as for initial IUD insertions.
- Recent exposure history or evidence of a purulent discharge from the cervix indicates referral for more detailed investigation at a genitourinary medicine (GUM) clinic. If *Chlamydia* is detected, the woman should be referred to a GUM service:
    - to be investigated for linked pathogens
    - to have necessary treatment and contact tracing arranged and
    - usually have the IUD insertion postponed.
- However, NHS resources can be saved by *not doing* unnecessary testing for vaginal organisms. To quote the FSRH guidance, '*in asymptomatic women . . . there is no indication to test or treat other lower genital tract organisms*'.
- In emergency contraception cases, screen—but treat anyway before the result is available (e.g. with azithromycin 1 g stat).
- The cervix should be cleansed (primarily physically, removing mucus by swabbing) before any device is inserted, with minimum trauma, following the manufacturer's instructions.
- In addition to the routine 6-week follow-up visit, the woman should be given clear details of the relevant symptoms of PID, and instructed as routine to telephone the practice nurse about 1 week post-insertion. This should identify any women with an early infection (during the crucial 20 post-insertion days of Fig. 16).

The *Chlamydia* screen can of course be omitted if, for example, the woman is over 35 years of age and the sexual history of 'mutual' monogamy is strong, particularly if her family is considered complete.

'Blind' prescription of an appropriate antibiotic is necessary in emergency cases, but the screening should still be done.

Otherwise, contact tracing is impossible and re-infection will simply occur later, the woman becoming one of the regular weekly cases that happen later than the first 20 days (Fig. 16).

Actinomyces-like organisms

These are sometimes reported in cervical smears—more commonly with long duration of use of either IUDs or IUSs.

If *Actinomyces*-like organisms (ALOs) are reported:

A First, call the woman for an extra consultation and examination, particularly bimanually. If all is normal, see below. But:

- If there are relevant symptoms or signs (pain, dyspareunia, excessive discharge, tenderness or any suggestion of an adnexal mass), an ultrasound scan should then be arranged, with a low threshold for gynaecological referral.
- After preliminary discussion with the microbiologist, the device should be removed and sent for culture. Treatment will have to be vigorous, usually prolonged, if frank pelvic actinomycosis is actually confirmed—it is a potentially life-threatening and fertility-destroying condition, although very rare.

Much more usually, the ALO finding occurs in asymptomatic and physical-sign-free women—who stay that way. Over-reaction might cause more morbidity through pregnancy than through actinomycosis, given the latter's rarity.

Second part of protocol on detection of ALOs

When there are no positive clinical findings, in consultation with the woman, the clinician may decide between **either of the following approaches, B or C, which have some supporting evidence:** MPC study re B, Mao et al. *Contraception* 1984; 30:535–544.

B

- Simple removal with or without reinsertion, and without antibiotic treatment.
  Reinsertion is NOT advisable at/after menopause, see p. 171.
- Advise the woman, along with written reference material, about the relevant symptoms that should make her seek a doctor urgently and tell her/him that she recently had an IUD or IUS plus ALOs.
- Repeat a cervical smear after 3 months (it will nearly always be negative) with a re-check bimanual examination. Both smear-taking and IUD follow-up then revert to normal.

C

- Leave the IUD or IUS alone after the initial thorough and fully reassuring examination, backed if there is any doubt by a negative pelvic ultrasound scan.
- Advise the woman, and provide her as for B with written material, about the relevant symptoms that should make her seek a doctor urgently and tell her/him that she is being followed up with an IUD or IUS plus ALOs.
- Arrange follow-up [which now is not done routinely for IUDs or IUSs (p. 142)], initially at 6 months, including a check for symptoms and bimanual examination as indicated.

Is ectopic pregnancy caused by copper IUDs?

This is another IUD myth. The main cause of ectopics is previous tubal infection, with one or both tubes being damaged. The non-causative association with IUDs comes about because they are even more effective at preventing pregnancy in the uterus than in the tube.

Ectopic pregnancies are actually reduced in number, because very few sperm get through the copper-containing uterine fluids to reach an egg, so very few implantations can occur in any damaged tube. However, there are even fewer implantations in the uterus. Thus, in the observed ratio, the denominator of intrauterine pregnancies is reduced more than the numerator of ectopics. So ectopics are more likely to be seen among the much-reduced number of IUD pregnancies—even though both types of pregnancy are actually reduced in frequency.

The estimated rate of ectopic pregnancy for sexually active Swedish women seeking pregnancy is 1.2 to 1.6 per 100 woman-years. The risk in users of either the T-Safe Cu 380A and its clones or of the LNG-IUS is estimated as 0.02 per 100 woman-years, which is at least 60 times lower, confirming the above argument.

Accordingly, UKMEC classifies a past history of ectopic pregnancy as WHO 1. Clinically, however, some caution is still necessary:

IUD/IUS Slogan 6
Any device-user with pain and a late or unusually light period or irregular bleeding has an ectopic pregnancy until proved otherwise.

Moreover, since there are even better anovulant options (e.g. COC, Cerazette™ or DMPA), *in nulliparae* I continue to view an actual past history of ectopic pregnancy as a relative contraindication (WHO 3) to IUDs (see p. 138).

Pain and bleeding

As already stated in IUD Slogan 3 (p. 122), pain and bleeding in IUD-users signify a dangerous condition—until proved otherwise (and indeed in early days it may well prove to be reactive, especially in a nullipara, and respond well to analgesics). Besides excluding conditions such as infection or an ectopic pregnancy or miscarriage, consider malpositioning of the frame of an IUD, which can cause pain through uterine spasms. Beyond the first few post-insertion days, a well-located IUD rarely causes pain. The same is true for the IUS which, moreover, over time often reduces pre-existing uterine pain.

Copper devices can be ideal, like reversible sterilization, for well-selected women with light menses. They need to know that:

- the duration of bleeding may increase, usually by a mean of 1 day
- the measured volume of bleeding by about one-third(although this can be a hardly noticeable addition if the woman's normal periods are light, e.g. 20 mL increasing to 27 mL)

Bleeding problems usually settle with time. If they do not, it may be necessary to change the method of contraception—perhaps to the LNG-IUS (see below).

Drug treatments may reduce the loss, but are not very satisfactory in the long term. The most successful therapies are mefenamic acid 500 mg eight hourly (which can simultaneously help pain as well, and so is usually tried first) and tranexamic acid 1 to 1.5 g eight hourly.

Duration of use

Studies regularly show reduced rates of discontinuation with increasing duration of use—whether for expulsion, infection or pain and bleeding, or indeed pregnancy. Coupled with the fact that most IUD complications are insertion related, it is good news that the banded devices T-Safe Cu 380A and clones may be used for 10 years or longer.

Above the age of 40, the agreed policy, since a 1990 statement in the Lancet by the FPA and the predecessor body of the FSRH, is as follows:

IUD Slogan 7

Any copper device (even a copper-wire-only type) that has been fitted above the age of 40 may be used for the rest of reproductive life (in practice, till age 55; see p. 171).

It never needs replacement, even though not licensed for that long. For the duration of use of the LNG-IUS in various situations, see below.

THE LEVONORGESTREL-RELEASING INTRAUTERINE SYSTEM

A schematic of the LNG-IUS (Mirena^{TM}) is shown in Figure 17.

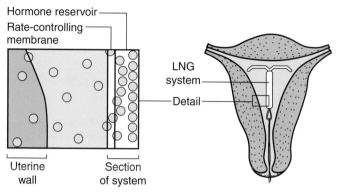

Figure 17
The levonorgestrel-releasing intrauterine system (LNG-IUS).

Method of action and effectiveness

LNG-IUS: the main points summarized

- It releases about 20 µg/24 hours of LNG from its polydimethyl-siloxane reservoir, through a rate-limiting membrane, for its licensed 5 years (and longer).
- Its main contraceptive effects are local, through changes to the cervical mucus and utero-tubal fluid that impair sperm migration, backed by endometrial changes impeding implantation.
- Its cumulative failure rate to 7 years was very low, at 1.1 per 100 women in the large Sivin study—even less to 5 years in a European multicentre trial by Anderson et al.
- Its efficacy is not detectably impaired by enzyme-inducing drugs.
- The systemic blood levels of LNG are initially higher (explaining early hormonal side effects) but fall in the first 3 months to under half of the mean levels in users of the LNG POP. For users, this can be explained as 'like taking three old-type POPs per week'. Hence, although ovarian function is altered in some women, especially in the first year, 85% show the ultrasound changes of normal ovulation.
- The amount of LNG in the blood is still enough to give unwanted hormone-type side effects in some women; otherwise, irregular light bleeding is the main problem.
- Even if they become amenorrhoeic—as many do, primarily through a local end-organ effect—in those who do not ovulate (as well as the majority who do), sufficient estrogen is produced for bone health.
- Return of fertility after removal is rapid, and appears to be complete.

Advantages and indications

The user of this method can expect the following advantages:

- A dramatic reduction in amount and, after the first few months (discussed below), duration of blood loss.
- Dysmenorrhoea is improved in most women.
- The LNG-IUS is the contraceptive method of choice for most women with heavy menstrual bleeding and it prevents/treats iron-deficiency anaemia. Indeed it should still be a first-line treatment when contraception is not needed, for both heavy bleeding and for menstrual pain (the latter even with normal blood loss).
- Endometriosis: gynaecologists now recognize the LNG-IUS as often ideal for long-term maintenance therapy, after initial diagnosis and treatment.
- Hormone-replacement therapy (HRT): by providing progestogenic protection of the uterus during estrogen replacement by any chosen route, the LNG-IUS uniquely, before final ovarian failure, offers 'forgettable, contraceptive, no-period and no PMS-type HRT'. For this increasingly popular indication, the LNG-IUS is currently licensed for 4 years before it must be replaced.
- Epilepsy: in a small series at the MPC, this was a very successful method for this condition, even in women on enzyme-inducer treatment.
- The LNG-IUS is, in short, a highly convenient and 'forgettable' contraceptive—with added gynaecological value.

The contraceptive advantages shown in the box above are, of course, shared with the T-Safe Cu 380A, which is the current gold standard for copper IUDs. However, this is where the similarity ends. The LNG-IUS fundamentally 'rewrites the textbooks' about IUDs, really only sharing the intrauterine location and certainly deserving a separate category (hence 'IUS').

What about infection/ectopic pregnancy risk and risk to future fertility?

Although IUDs do not themselves cause PID (see above), they fail to prevent it, and there is a suspicion that they sometimes worsen the attacks that occur. The LNG-IUS may actually reduce the frequency of clinical PID in long-term users, perhaps through the progestogenic effect on cervical mucus, particularly in the youngest age groups who are most at risk. However, the risk is certainly not eliminated and condom use should still be advocated. But the available data make it possible to offer the LNG-IUS to some young women requesting a 'forgettable' contraceptive who would not be good candidates for conventional copper IUDs. Their future fertility is most unlikely to be adversely affected.

The data published for this device show (like the banded copper IUDs) a massive reduction in ectopic risk, which can be attributed to its greater efficacy by the sperm-blocking mechanism that reduces the risk of pregnancy in any site. However, in the case of a past history of an ectopic pregnancy, an anovulant method would be even better.

Problems and disadvantages of the LNG-IUS

As with any IUD:
- Expulsion can occur, and there is the usual small risk of:
- Perforation, minimized by its 'withdrawal' as opposed to a 'plunger' technique of insertion.
- Pain suggests malpositioning: it is not expected, pain is usually improved with an IUS. Check by ultrasound scan, indeed ahead of insertion whenever fibroids are suspected at the preliminary examination.
- A significant problem is the high incidence in the first post-insertion months of uterine bleeding, which, although small in quantity, may be very frequent or continuous and can cause considerable inconvenience.
- In later months, amenorrhoea is commonly reported—sometimes perceived as a problem, though it is really not so!

Women can accept the early weeks of light bleeding, even if very frequent, as a worthwhile price to pay for all the other advantages of the method: provided they are well informed *in advance* of LNG-IUS fitting. They can be confident that perseverance will be rewarded, since this early problem has such a good prognosis.

The oligo-amenorrhoea that follows can be explained and interpreted to a woman as an advantage—gently debunking the myth that menstruation serves an excretory function—not an adverse side effect but a positive benefit of the method.

Women should also be forewarned that, although this method is mainly local in its action, it is not exclusively so. Therefore, there is a small incidence of 'hormonal' side effects such as bloatedness, acne and depression. These do usually improve, often within 2 months, in parallel with the known decline in the higher initial LNG blood levels. Strangely, in comparative studies such 'hormonal' symptoms have not actually been proved to occur more often than in copper IUD–users.

The frequency of developing functional ovarian cysts is also probably increased, although they are usually asymptomatic. If pain results, they should be investigated/monitored, but they usually resolve spontaneously.

Contraindications

Many of the contraindications of this method are shared with copper IUDs (see below). The additional few that are unique to LNG-IUS are due to the actions of its LNG hormone, of which some gets into the systemic circulation, and are discussed in the following box.

Unique contraindications (WHO group as stated) for the LNG-IUS, among intrauterine methods

- Current breast cancer—this is WHO 4 according to UKMEC, with the LNG-IUS becoming usable on a WHO 3 basis after 5 years' remission, like all the other progestogen-only methods. In my view:
  - since the LNG-IUS gives the lowest overall systemic hormone dose of such methods, and
  - given the suggestive data that it may protect against tamoxifen-induced pre-cancer changes in the endometrium, in selected cases this WHO 3 status might be agreed considerably sooner, after consultation with the oncologist
- Trophoblastic disease (any)—this is WHO 4 while blood hCG levels are high, but there is no problem (WHO 1) after full recovery (hCG undetectable)
- Current liver tumour or severe (decompensated) hepatocellular disease (WHO 3) or past CHC-related cholestasis (WHO 2)
- Gallbladder disease (WHO 2)
- Current severe active arterial or venous thrombotic disease, risk factors or predispositions (all WHO 2)

In addition, the LNG-IUS should not be used as a post-coital intrauterine contraceptive (failures have been reported); acting by a hormone, it appears not to act as rapidly as the intrauterine copper ion does.

Duration of use of the LNG-IUS in the older woman

The product is licensed for 5 years
However, it should be noted:
- For contraception, effective use is evidence based but unlicensed for up to 7 years. For a woman under age 40, because of her greater fertility, replacement after the usual 5 years would be advisable. But the older woman whose LNG-IUS was fitted above the age of say 40 might continue for 7 years, at her fully empowered request (but always on a 'named-patient' basis—pp. 173–5). Furthermore, the FSRH guidance (2007) states that women who have the LNG-IUS inserted at the age of *45 years* or over for contraception can retain the device until the menopause is confirmed or contraception is no longer required (see Slogan 8).
- As part of HRT, current practice for safe endometrial protection would be to change it at 4 years, though the data support and other countries permit 5 years.
- But if the LNG-IUS is not being and will not be used for either contraception or HRT, it could be left in situ for as long as it continues to work, in the control of heavy and/or painful uterine bleeding, and then removed after ovarian failure can be finally assured. However, it should not normally be in situ beyond about age 55 (actinomycosis risk, see p. 171).

IUS Slogan 8
Women who have the LNG-IUS inserted at the age of 45 years or over for contraception can retain the device until the menopause is confirmed, or until contraception is no longer required—possibly up to age 55 in fact (see p. 171).

Conclusions—the LNG-IUS

This method fulfils many of the accepted criteria for an ideal contraceptive (see the box on p. 8). It approaches 100%

reversibility, effectiveness and even, after some delay, convenience. This is because, after the initial months of frequent uterine bleedings and spotting, the usual outcomes of either intermittent light menses or amenorrhoea are very acceptable to most women. Adverse side effects are few and, in general, they are in the 'nuisance' category rather than hazardous.

However, this method does fail on some criteria: above all that it is not sufficiently protective against STIs, especially the sexually transmitted viruses, so wherever STI transmission risk applies condoms must be used in addition. We also eagerly await an implantable version, based on the GyneFix concept.

CONTRAINDICATIONS TO INTRAUTERINE CONTRACEPTION—GENERALLY

Note that these apply primarily to copper IUDs but also to the LNG-IUS, except where stated. (The contraindications that are unique to the IUS have already been listed.)

Absolute—but perhaps temporary—contraindications (WHO 4) to fitting all IUDs and the LNG-IUS

- Suspicion of pregnancy
- Undiagnosed irregular genital tract bleeding, till cause known/ treated as necessary
- Significant current infection: post-septic abortion, current pelvic infection or STI, undiagnosed pelvic tenderness/deep dyspareunia or purulent cervical discharge
- Significant immunosuppression
- Malignant or benign trophoblastic disease, while hCG is abnormal (UKMEC 4 for IUDs and the IUS, according to UKMEC). This is in case the uterine wall is invaded by tumour, increasing the risk of a perforation. But this becomes WHO 1 when hCG is undetectable
- (LNG-IUS only) Breast cancer is UKMEC 4, becoming UKMEC 3 in remission (see p. 84). However, this might be an indication for a copper IUD
- The woman's own ethics forbidding her to use a method with a possible post-fertilization mechanism (pp. 145–6)

Absolute permanent contraindications (WHO 4) to fitting IUDs/ LNG-IUS

- Markedly distorted uterine cavity, or cavity sounding to less than 5.5 cm depth (but this is only WHO 2 for GyneFix)
- Known true allergy to a constituent of the device
- Wilson's disease (copper IUDs only—this is precautionary advice, through absent data)
- Pulmonary hypertension, because of a risk of a fatal vasovagal reaction through cervical instrumentation

Note that previous endocarditis and risk thereof are WHO 1, NOT now considered contraindications, nor is any antibiotic cover required for IUD or IUS insertions (see BNF Section 5.1).

Relative contraindications to intrauterine contraceptives—WHO 2 unless otherwise stated

This is a longish list, but in all cases meaning an IUD or especially the LNG-IUS is usable, with some degree of caution.

1. Nulliparity and young age, especially less than 20 years. This combination is WHO 2 because the actual insertion process is likely to be more difficult, and there are more serious implications should there be a severe infection (with no babies yet). But WHO 2 does mean 'broadly usable'. Moreover, UKMEC classifies nulliparity above age 20 as WHO 1 for both copper IUDs (often inserted as emergency contraception, see next chapter) and the IUS.

2. Lifestyle of self or partner(s) at high risk of STIs, or past history of pelvic infection. Combined with (1) this may equate to WHO 3: if the method is even so chosen, there needs to be committed condom use.

3. Recent exposure to high risk of a STI (e.g. after rape). As emergency contraception, a copper IUD may be used (WHO 2) with full antibiotic cover (and after *Chlamydia* testing done).

4. Known HIV infection. While controlled by drug therapy, this is only WHO 2. LNG-IUS is better still because of reduced blood loss (added condom use is routinely advised anyway).

5. Past history of ectopic pregnancy or other history suggesting high ectopic risk *in a nullipara* is WHO 3, in my view (UKMEC is less cautious), but WHO 1 (as UKMEC) if there are living children. If used, banded copper IUDs or IUS are the best; but it is even better to use an anovulant method.

6. Suspected subfertility already. This is WHO 2 for any cause, or WHO 3 if it relates to a tubal cause.

7. Post-partum, between 48 hours and 4 weeks (excess risk of perforation; WHO 3).
8. Fibroids or congenital abnormality of the uterus with some but not marked distortion of the uterine cavity (see above). This is WHO 2 for framed IUDs or IUSs, WHO 1 for GyneFix (if inserted by an expert, as perforation risk high when cavity distorted).
9. Severely scarred or distorted uterus, e.g. after myomectomy (WHO 3).
10. After endometrial ablation/resection—there is a risk of the IUD becoming stuck in the shrunken and scarred cavity. LNG-IUS or GyneFix are usable in selected cases.
11. Heavy periods, with or without anaemia before insertion for any reason, including anticoagulation. This is an indication for the LNG-IUS (WHO 1).
12. Dysmenorrhoea, any type. The LNG-IUS may well benefit all types, can indeed be used to treat pain in the absence of heaviness of bleeding.
13. Endometriosis. This may be benefited by the LNG-IUS (WHO 1), to help local symptoms in addition to systemic treatment.
14. Previous perforation of uterus. This is WHO 2, almost WHO 1, at least for the small defect in the uterine fundus after a previous IUD perforation. Healing is so complete that it is usually difficult even to locate the site of the previous event.
15. Pelvic tuberculosis is WHO 3, WHO 4 if future fertility is hoped for.

Notes
- If it is available and a copper IUD is desired, GyneFix, being frameless, would often be preferable for (8), (9) and (10).
- The LNG-IUS may be preferred or *indicated,* notably for the conditions listed in (4) and (10)–(13).

COUNSELLING, INSERTION AND FOLLOW-UP

Timing of insertions—for all intrauterine contraceptives

Generally
- In the normal cycle, timing must be planned to avoid an already implanted pregnancy, but otherwise it is a myth that insertion is best during menses (higher expulsion rates are reported then, in fact).

- With copper IUDs (because they are such efficient post-coital methods), insertion can be at any time up to 5 days after the calculated day of ovulation, or even:
- At any time in the cycle—if the provider is reasonably certain of the woman not being, nor just about to be, pregnant in a conception cycle (see p. 166).
- For the LNG-IUS, a more cautious timing policy is advised (see below).
- Post-partum insertions of IUDs or IUSs are usually at 6 weeks and acceptable from 4 weeks (beware the reported increased risk of perforation). If the woman is not fully breastfeeding, conception risk should be discussed (pp. 167–9)—and with the IUS, additional contraception is advised for 7 days.
- Following first-trimester abortion (but only after preliminary counselling and with full agreement by the woman), immediate insertion has been established—by systematic reviews and good studies—to be good practice (see slogan below). This means the immediate insertion being:
  – On the day of surgical-induced abortion or (more controversially) the second part of a medical abortion, if the uterus is clearly empty—this can be checked by on-the-spot ultrasound.

IUD/IUS Slogan 9—regarding pregnancy termination

If an intrauterine method is accepted for future contraception, the *immediate insertion* of an IUD or IUS should be encouraged as the *normal*, default thing to do, after pregnancy termination.

Additional points about insertion timing for the LNG-IUS

- In the normal cycle: Insertion for the IUS should be no later than day 7 of the normal cycle, since it does not operate as an effective post-coital contraceptive and because, in addition, any fetus might be harmed by conception in the first cycle (since there are known to be extremely high local LNG concentrations in the endometrium). Later insertion is acceptable, but only if there has been believable abstinence beforehand and with continued contraception (e.g. condoms) post insertion, for 7 days.
- If a woman is on a CHC or POP/Cerazette or Nexplanon or DMPA: the IUS can normally be inserted any time, with no added precautions. This is often ideal (see below).

Clinical implications

As for Nexplanon, insertions only in the above tiny natural-cycle window are a logistic and conception risk nightmare! So a useful practical tip is to actively recommend at counselling, as normal routine, the use of an anovulant method (usually a CHC or Cerazette), for use from then until the LNG-IUS insertion. Insertion can then be at any convenient time, without any timing problems or conception anxiety. If the woman has amenorrhoea through her previous method (e.g. on DMPA), there is also a *suggestion* that early bleeding problems with the IUS may be minimized—but this needs more study.

Good analgesia is crucial—more practical tips

- Pre-medication with a prostaglandin inhibitor while waiting for the procedure should be routine for all insertions. An MPC trial of mefenamic acid 500 mg given about 40 minutes beforehand reported (1980) a statistically significant reduction in the 'cramping' variety of delayed pain with the former, but it did not help the immediate 'sharp' pains from the cervix (see next bullet).
- There is a very unpredictable but sometimes bad pain that any woman (even a relaxed parous woman) may experience, caused by the application of the tenaculum at 12 o'clock on the cervix; and an initial 1-mL dose of 1% lidocaine injected 2 to 3 minutes ahead completely abolishes this. So it is my practice to offer this to all-comers.
- Full local anaesthesia by para-cervical block should be more often offered as a choice. It should almost always be used if the cervix has to be dilated above Hegar 5 or the uterine cavity explored.
- A relaxed ambience, with an assistant present and with both providers using what has been termed 'vocal local' reduces both anxiety and pain . . ..
- Topical lidocaine gel may also help, if applied far enough ahead.

Counselling and follow-up

After considering the contraindications, there should be an unhurried discussion of all the main practical points about this method with the woman, focusing on infection risk and the importance of reporting pain as a symptom at any time—and of telephoning if it occurs in the early weeks post insertion.

The pre-insertion examination should usually include a *Chlamydia* screen (p. 127), and she should always be given a user-friendly backup leaflet. She should be assured that during the use of the method, in the event of relevant symptoms or if she can no longer feel her threads, she will always receive prompt advice ('open house') and, as indicated, a pelvic examination.

The only important routine follow-up is the visit at about 6 weeks after insertion. This is to:

- discuss with the woman any menstrual (or other) symptoms
- check for expulsion, including partial expulsion: the overall rate is about 4% to 5% with all framed IUDs and the IUS, mainly in the first 3 months
- exclude infection, i.e. no relevant symptoms, tenderness or mass

---

IUD/IUS Slogan 10—regarding follow-up
With IUDs and the IUS, until the first follow-up visit has happened, the insertion cannot be said to be complete.

Afterwards the woman should be advised of the 'open house' policy, meaning *she will not need to be seen routinely* but will always get prompt help if she has symptoms as given in the box below.

Reasons for an IUD- or IUS-user seeking urgent medical assistance:

- Pelvic pain, low central or one-sided
- Deep dyspareunia
- Much increased or offensive discharge
- Missed period
- Significant menstrual abnormalities
- Non-palpable threads (if could previously feel them) or overt expulsion
- She or partner can feel the stem of partially expelled device

---

Training for the actual insertion process

A book like this is not the right medium for teaching insertion techniques. The FSRH training leading to the Letter of Competence in intrauterine contraception techniques is strongly recommended. This starts with e-learning on e-SRH, followed by further self-directed theoretical training to complete the e-SRH Module 18—and then practical training using a model uterus and culminating with at least seven competent insertions of copper IUDs and the IUS. Full details are at www.fsrh.org/pdfs/FormT.pdf.

As we have already noted, it is worth getting all aspects of insertion training right, given the truth of **IUD Slogan 1** (p. 119)—that *Insertion can be a factor in the causation of almost every category of IUD problems*. The trainee's expertise must also be maintained thereafter through the FSRH's recommended minimum of one IUD insertion per month, on average.

Emergency contraception

There are two basic varieties of emergency contraception (EC), initiated after unprotected sexual intercourse (UPSI):

- Copper ions, inserted as a copper IUD
- Hormonal methods, taken by mouth

Among the latter, past methods included estrogens alone in very high dose and the combined oral emergency contraceptive (COEC) using LNG 500 μg + EE 100 μg repeated in 12 hours. Currently marketed hormonal EC methods in the United Kingdom are

- the levonorgestrel progestogen-only emergency contraceptive (LNG EC, Levonelle 1500™ or Levonelle One Step™) in a stat dose of LNG 1500 μg and
- ulipristal acetate (UPA, ellaOne™) in a dose of 30 mg.

These are discussed below (pp. 147–152).

The latest Faculty Guidance on emergency contraception can be found at:
www.fsrh.org/pdfs/CEUguidanceEmergencyContraception11.pdf

COMBINED ORAL EMERGENCY CONTRACEPTION

Though no longer marketed in the United Kingdom as such, it is a useful though little-known fact that this one can be *constructed* using the standard LNG 150 μg + EE 30 μg COC, which has at least 60 names and is marketed in almost every country on the planet. WHO advises four tablets of, for example, Microgynon 30™ stat up to 72 hours after UPSI, repeated in 12 hours. It is rather sad to think of the number of women worldwide having unwanted conceptions due to ignorance in their society (and among providers) of this simple option, which they would have wanted to use.

COPPER INTRAUTERINE DEVICES

Mechanism of action

Insertion of a copper IUD—not the LNG IUS (see p. 136)—before implantation is the most effective EC method available. Copper ions are immediately toxic to sperm and also prevent implantation. This means, after consultation with the woman, that insertion may proceed *in good faith*:

- up to 5 days after the first sexual exposure (regardless of cycle length); **and also**
- up to 5 days after the (earliest) calculated ovulation day.

This means working out, together with her:

- the soonest likely next menstrual start day, then
- subtracting 14 days for the mean life of the corpus luteum, and
- adding 5 days to allow for the shortest estimated interval from fertilization to implantation.
  See discussion on this in FSRH Guidance 2012.

The judge's summing up in a 1991 Court Case (Regina vs. Dhingra) gives legal support to thus intervening up to 5 days post-ovulation/fertilization:

> *I further hold ... that a pregnancy cannot come into existence until the fertilized ovum has become implanted in the womb, and that that stage is not reached until, at the earliest, the 20th day of a normal 28 day cycle ...*

Moreover, the UK fpa convened a Judicial Review of Emergency Contraception which also confirmed in 2002 the long-held position of most ethicists who considered the matter—namely that a pregnancy begins at implantation, not when an egg is fertilized—and gave this concept legal status in the United Kingdom. However, some women as well as a few providers believe that any intervention after fertilization constitutes abortion not contraception. That view must be respected and allowed for in consultations (including of course re long-term use of the IUD or IUS, p. 137).

Effectiveness of copper as EC

The copper IUD prevents conception in well over 99% of women who present, or over 98% of those who might be expected otherwise to conceive, even in cases of multiple exposure since the last menstrual period. Women who present almost always prefer an oral method, but in some circumstances may need to be encouraged to consider this instead:

Indications for EC by copper IUD

In selected individuals, IUD insertion may be preferable to oral EC:

- When maximum efficacy is the woman's priority—her choice. UKMEC says it should be offered to all—indeed, even to those presenting within 72 hours.
- When exposure occurred more than 72 hours earlier, or in cases of multiple exposure: insertion may be
  – up to 5 days after the earliest UPSI at any time in the cycle, or
  – if there have been many UPSI acts, no later than 5 days after calculated ovulation (p. 145).
- In many women—often, though not always, parous—when it is to be retained as their long-term method*. Always try to insert a banded IUD (e.g. the Mini TT 380 Slimline) when long-term use is likely.
- In the presence of contraindications to the hormonal method [unusual, but enzyme-inducer drugs are an example (WHO 3)—so consider an IUD, e.g. a St John's Wort user].
- If the woman is coincidentally suffering a vomiting attack when she presents, or unexpectedly and repeatedly vomits her dose of hormonal EC within 2 hours (for UPA, the SPC says within 3 hours), in a case with particularly high pregnancy risk.

*Yet it may be appropriate, in many young women when one of the other bullets apply, to remove the IUD after their next menses—when the 'emergency' is over and they are established on a new method, such as the COC or injectable or implant.

Contraindications to the IUD method and clinical implications

The IUD method has a number of recognized contraindications (pp. 137–9) and always risks short-term pain, bleeding or post-insertion infection, not to mention the inevitable 'hassle'. So this option needs to be provided well, despite the 'emergency'.

A good sexual history (see p. 7) should be taken from everyone presenting for EC, and UK studies suggest an above-average risk that such women are carrying *Chlamydia trachomatis*. If the sexual history is confirmatory and the woman agrees (after explaining, as one always should, the relationship implications of the test if positive), she should be tested at least for this STI—even if having hormonal EC. Warn also that recently acquired STIs may not be detectable till later retesting. The result not being available pre-IUD insertion, there should be

- prophylactic antibiotic cover, e.g. with azithromycin 1 g stat and
- arrangements for contact tracing to follow if STI test results later prove positive.

Insertion might be expected to be difficult sometimes, especially but not exclusively in nulliparae: but helpfully this rarely needs to be on the day of presentation. It can usually be arranged later after referral to a skilled colleague at a nearby service, given the ability to use IUDs later in the cycle, up to 5 days after ovulation (see above). Insertion could be on day 18, say, for a woman with a 27-day shortest cycle, presenting at a branch surgery on day 15 after high-risk UPSI repeatedly prior to that.

In such cases, UKMEC recommends giving hormonal EC on the day of presentation, as a holding manoeuvre.

HORMONAL EMERGENCY CONTRACEPTION

After sexual exposure, the earlier the treatment is given, the better—according to some but not all the studies. Yet EC remains a better lay term than 'morning-after Pill', since it leaves open the facts—see box on next page:

Levonorgestrel emergency contraception

Dose: LNG 1500 μg stat within 72 hours of sexual exposure

Mechanism of action

Given at or before ovulation, the method

- interferes with follicle development, either inhibiting altogether or possibly delaying ovulation—*clinically,* impress therefore on any user the continuing conception risk from unprotected sex post-treatment;
- makes the cervical mucus hostile to sperm.

However, given later in a cycle, after fertilization, it is now thought to have an almost negligible effect to prevent implantation. If there is thought to be the need for that mechanism, the most effective agent remains the copper ion.

Effectiveness and advantages of LNG EC

Main advantages of LNG EC in comparison with the former COEC method:
- Greater effectiveness when treatment began within 24 hours of a single exposure—in the circumstances of the 1998 WHO trial
- Reduced rates of the main side effects of nausea and vomiting
- In ordinary practice, virtually no contraindications

The apparent effectiveness of LNG EC with treatment up to 72 hours after a single sexual exposure in the WHO Study was around 99%—but this represents prevention of only 70% to 75% of the expected pregnancies, since most of those who present would not actually have conceived. Moreover, in the real world, multiple acts of UPSI without 'perfect' condom use both before and after the treatment can greatly increase the conception risk. This may be reducible by giving LNG EC more than once (in the same cycle)—which is endorsed by the FSRH though not as yet licensed.

Emergency contraception with ulipristal acetate

Dose: UA as ellaOne™ (HRA Pharma) 30 mg stat within 120 hours (5 days) of sexual exposure

Mechanism of action

It contains UPA which is a synthetic selective progesterone receptor modulator with antagonist and partial agonist effects. It therefore prevents progesterone from occupying its receptors, including in the endometrium. It is *also* established as a more potent inhibitor of ovulation than LNG EC (as Levonelle 1500).

Effectiveness

In a meta-analysis of two studies, UPA prevented around twice as many pregnancies as LNG, and the best current estimate of actual conceptions prevented is c. 85%. It also has sustained efficacy over time beyond 72 hours through till 120 hours after the earliest UPSI in that cycle. Hence, unlike LNG EC, it is fully licensed for use until then, 5 days after sex.

However,

- UPA is not recommended for use more than once per cycle – an accepted though unlicensed practice with LNG EC. There is no evidence of any kind of harm if LNG is inadvertently given to an implanted pregnancy, not (so far) established as true with UPA.
- It is more expensive for the NHS, though this has been shown to be cost effective, primarily by preventing more conceptions.
- Users need pre-warning that around 20% of women in clinical trials reported a delay of 7 or more days in their next menses after use of UPA, *even when conception prevented*.

Effect on other hormones

- UPA, by its progestogen receptor antagonist effect, may until it has been excreted reduce the effectiveness of any progestogen-containing contraceptives. If therefore any POP (e.g.

Cerazette™) or any CHC with progestogen is to be (re)-started immediately, this might be a reason to choose LNG EC.

- If UPA is preferred, pending more data HRA Pharma advises additional precautions with the new hormonal method till the next period. Since the half-life of UPA is only 32.4 hours, in the absence of definitive studies the FSRH has proposed that 7 days of additional precautions is sufficient (i.e. 7 days *more than the advice normally given when quick-starting* that hormonal method). This means in effect 7 + 7 = 14 days for CHCs and 7 + 2 = 9 days for POPs.

Maintenance of efficacy

Enzyme-inducer drug (EID) treatment

If the woman is taking any one of these (listed on pp. 55–6, including St John's Wort; also bosentan p. 82), hormonal EC is WHO 3. As usual, this category means that it would be much better to use an alternative, in this case

- insertion of a copper IUD (completely unaffected by drugs).

If not acceptable, the choice is either

- LNG EC with the dose of LNG EC being doubled, i.e. two tablets totalling 3 mg stat [unlicensed use (pp. 173–5)—but endorsed by the FSRH] or, in my view,
- UPA with the dose doubled to 60 mg stat. This is a biologically plausible but similarly unlicensed practice, and we need more clinical data. It is not yet (2012) endorsed by the FSRH.

Contraindications to either brand of hormonal EC

There are vanishingly few WHO 4 conditions:
Aside from current pregnancy when it would be redundant anyway, in my view these are
- known *severe* allergy to a constituent (moderate/dubious allergy would be WHO 3)
- known *acute* porphyria (WHO 3), though with greater reluctance (close to WHO 4) if history of severe attack(s) induced by sex hormones. UKMEC says WHO 2, but my view is more cautious

- if it emerges on discussion that the woman's own ethics preclude intervention post-coitally (or more relevantly, post-fertilization)— i.e. she disagrees with the UK legal view (see above)
- for UPA (until more data): avoid concurrent use with systemic medicines that increase gastric pH: absorption may be impaired
- UPA is also not currently recommended with severe hepatic impairment nor with asthma poorly controlled by oral glucocorticoids

---

Relative contraindications (WHO 3 or 2)
- Enzyme-inducer drug treatment, see above (WHO 3)—copper IUD preferred
- Current breast cancer (WHO 2 due to uncertainty, but an adverse effect is unlikely with such short exposure)
- If a significant absorption problem is anticipated (WHO 2, or WHO 4 during acute vomiting, see above)

Breastfeeding is not a contraindication, although the conception risk is of course usually (p. 80; p. 164) so low that EC treatment would rarely be needed. If it is indicated, the infant should not be harmed in any way by the tiny amount of either LNG or UPA reaching the milk. (The SPC for UPA also advises no breastfeeds for 36 hours).

WHICH EC METHOD TO USE?

The FSRH Guidance of August 2012 states clearly that providers "should...inform women about the different methods with regard to efficacy, adverse effects, interactions, medical eligibility and need for additional contraceptive precautions. The efficacy of UPA has been demonstrated up to 120 hours *and can be offered to all eligible women requesting EC during this time period* [JG's emphasis]. It is the only oral EC licensed for use between 72 and 120 hours. If [any provider] is unable to provide a method of EC, local referral mechanisms should facilitate timely access to a service that can provide the woman's preferred method."

Any other idications? As we have seen, if it appears that EC will be given during the approx 5 days between fertilization and implantation, *the most effective course despite the perceived 'hassle' for all concerned is always copper IUD insertion*. But could UPA with its anti-progestogen activity be a new option here, so long as it is made very clear that it is *definitely less effective* than copper? This use based on the calculated ovulation day is controversial, clearly unlicensed, and is not advised by HRA Pharma nor, as yet, by the FSRH. Also, it is a 'black triangle' drug, so beware, if used thus the guidance at pp. 173–5 must be followed to the letter. Moreover, it should be recorded that the woman clearly understands that there is some doubt re UPA's effectiveness at blocking implantation and, unlike LNG, re its safety for a pregnancy if, inadvertently, it were given after one had implanted.

SUMMARY: COUNSELLING AND MANAGEMENT OF EC CASES

First, evaluate the possibility of sexual abuse or rape. Then, **in a context that preserves confidentiality**—and feels that way to the client—using (crucially) a good leaflet, such as that of the fpa, as the basis for discussion, help the woman to make a fully informed and autonomous choice. This could be any of the *three* EC methods, or, for some cases who present too late, taking no action at all (i.e. waiting 'with fingers crossed' for the next period).

Pharmacists should ensure privacy for the discussion and have a low threshold to refer all cases outside their specified remit to an appropriate clinical provider [e.g. because more suitable for UPA—unless there are local PGD arrangements or it becomes licensed for direct sales—or for a copper IUD].

Clinical management

- Careful assessment of *menstrual/coital history* is essential. Probe for other exposures to risk earlier than the one presented with. Note: Ovulation is such a variable event and LNG EC and UPA are so safe that most women are best treated whenever they present—in the 'normal' cycle.
- *Assess contraindications.* The mode of action may itself pose the only contraindication/problem, for some individuals. It may sometimes be appreciated by a woman who has these ethical concerns that LNG EC, despite being after sex, is now known to have negligible effects after fertilization. This EC method might be even more acceptable if it is clearly going to be given well before ovulation in a given cycle and she can be sure it will be out of her body by the time of implantation.

- *Medical risks* may be a concern, and should be set out in the information leaflet that is given, especially:
  - *The failure rate*: remind the woman that the figures relate to a single exposure. The failure rate is close to nil for the IUD.
  - *Teratogenicity* if there is a failure: this is believed to be negligible if EC hormones are given as they should be before implantation, since they cannot reach the unimplanted blastocyst in sufficient concentration to cause any effect. Follow-up of women who have kept their pregnancies has so far not shown any increased risk of major abnormalities above the background rate of 2%, though data on UPA failures are scanty.
  - *Ectopic pregnancy*: if this follows after either hormonal or copper EC, as it may, the EC was not causative. It can only occur in a pre-existing damaged tube and would have happened anyway, with or without this (pre-implantation) treatment. However, a clear past history of ectopic pregnancy or pelvic infection remains a reason for specific forewarning with any EC method, and **all** women should be warned to report back urgently if they get **pain**. Also, providers must 'think ectopic' whenever EC by hormones or by copper may have failed, or there is an unusual bleeding pattern post-treatment.
- *Side effects:*
  - *With LNG EC* in the WHO 2002 trial, nausea occurred in 15% and vomiting in 1.4% of users. If the contraceptive dose is vomited within 2 hours, before resorting to an IUD the woman may be given a further tablet with an anti-emetic: the best seems to be domperidone (Motilium) 10 mg.
  - *With UPA*, in the RCT comparing with LNG EC (Glasier *et al Lancet* 2010; **375**: 555–562), all reported symptoms were similar (eg vomiting 1.5%), with no statistical differences.

- *Future contraception*, both in the current cycle (in case the LNG EC or UPA merely postpone ovulation)—often condoms—and in the long term, should be discussed. The IUD option covers both aspects (for a suitable long-term user). Inform the woman that using EC every month is not advised: by the end of a year there is a higher risk of failure that way than by regular use of almost any approved method. If the COC or injectable is chosen, it should normally be started as soon as the woman is convinced her next period is normal—usually on the first or second day— without the need for additional contraception thereafter.
- But 'Quick start' *of almost any of the 'medical' contraceptives* is also an option in selected cases. This means starting the long-term method immediately after the EC (pp.167–8), along with the approved advice for added condom use. If UPA was the EC method, this should be for 7 days longer than usually advised (pp. 149–50).

Follow-up should be no less than 3 weeks after the last UPSI, for a hopefully negative pregnancy test. In these cases the clinician must be confident that the benefits (especially the greater probability of future compliance) outweigh the conception risks. 'Quick start' is unlicensed, so records should be meticulous as described at pp. 173–5, with appropriate documented warnings.

The above description highlights the importance of a good rapport to obtain an honest and accurate coital/menstrual history and to promote more effective contraception in future.

FOLLOW-UP

Women receiving LNG EC or UPA (except with 'Quick start') rarely need to be seen again routinely, but should be instructed to return

- if they experience pain, or
- their expected period is *more than 7 days late*, or lighter than usual.

IUD-acceptors return usually in 4 to 6 weeks for a routine check-up; or perhaps for device removal, once established on what for them is a more appropriate long-term method.

SPECIAL INDICATIONS FOR EC

These apply to coital exposure when the following have occurred:

- **Omission of anything more than two COC tablets after the PFI**, or of more than two Pills in the first seven in the packet—see p. 49. As explained there, after the first Pill-taking week, since seven tablets have been taken to render the ovaries quiescent, Pill-omissions almost never indicate emergency treatment. Moreover, towards the end of a packet (Pill-days 15–21), simple omission of the next PFI will always suffice—no matter how many Pills have been missed, up to seven (which is of course routine in that normal PFI week!).
- **Delay in taking a POP tablet for more than 3 hours**, outside of lactation, implying loss of the mucus effect, followed by sexual exposure before mucus-based contraception was

restored (presumed in 2 days—p. 79). The POP is restarted immediately after the emergency regimen, 2 days of added precautions are advised, and follow-up agreed. EC is more rarely required for missed Cerazette tablets (see p. 80).

- **If the POP-user (or Cerazette-user) is breastfeeding,** EC would only be indicated if either the breastfeeding or the POP-taking were unusually inadequate (p. 80)!

- **Removal or expulsion of an IUD** before the time of implantation, if another IUD cannot be inserted, for some reason.

- **Further exposure in the same natural cycle**—e.g. due to failure of barrier contraception more than 1 day after a dose of EC has been taken. Additional courses of LNG EC are supported by the FSRH, 'if clinically indicated', given reasonable precautions to avoid treating after implantation (yet repeated use thereafter will not induce an abortion). This use is, again, outside the terms of the licence (see pp. 173–5). Repeated use of UPA in this way is not currently advised.

- **Use of UPA, not LNG EC, up to 5 days after the calculated ovulation day,** regardless of the number of unprotected sexual acts up to that time.
  This controversial as well as unlicensed indication was discussed above. Women should be told of the limited evidence of efficacy—and also that a copper IUD would definitely be more effective.

- **Overdue injections of DMPA with continuing sexual intercourse.** See p. 94 re when this might be appropriate.

- **Advanced provision of hormonal EC**: The FSRH supports this in selected cases, to increase early use when required— e.g. when travelling abroad to cover the possibility of UPSI through condom non-use or rupture (or even rape).

In all circumstances of use of EC, the women should be aware (as stated in the fpa leaflet) that
- The method might fail.
- It is not an abortifacient.
- It is given too soon to be able to harm a baby.

Other reversible methods*

BARRIER METHODS

Barrier methods are not yet out of fashion! In spite of well-known disadvantages, they all (above all condoms) can provide useful protection against STIs. *All users of this type of method should be informed about EC, in case of lack of use or failure in use.* Guidance documents are available, see www.fsrh.org

Vegetable- and oil-based lubricants, and the bases for many prescribable vaginal products, can seriously damage and lead to rupture of rubber: baby oil destroys up to 95% of a condom's strength within 15 minutes. Beware of ad hoc use of, or contamination by, substances from the kitchen or bathroom cupboard! The box on p. 157 lists some common vaginal preparations that should be regarded as unsafe to use with rubber condoms and diaphragms—but it is not a complete list. Water-based products such as KY Jelly, and also glycerine and silicone lubricants, do not harm latex, but all oils and creams should be regarded as suspect.

This problem does not affect plastic condoms such as Avanti Ultima, Mates Skyn and Pasante Unique. However, there is no evidence that any of these is less likely to rupture for mechanical reasons.

---

*Male and female sterilization—especially the former, which is more effective—are useful options for some couples, but not reversible so not within the remit of this particular book.

Condoms

Condoms are the only proven barrier to transmission of HIV—yet, at the time of writing, it still remains impossible in the United Kingdom for most couples to obtain this life-saver free of charge from every GP. Condoms are second in usage to the Pill among those under the age of 30 and to sterilization above that age.

One GP has reported a failure rate as low as 0.4 per 100 woman-years, but 2 to 15 is more representative. Failure, often unrecognized at the time, can almost always be attributed to incorrect use—mainly through escape of a small amount of semen either before or after the main ejaculation. Conceptions—particularly among the young or those who have become a bit casual after years of using a simple method such as the COC—can sometimes be 'iatrogenic' simply because of lack of explanation of the basics by a clinician or pharmacist.

Some users are entirely satisfied with the condom, whereas others use it as a temporary or backup method. For many who have become accustomed to alternatives not related to intercourse, it is completely unacceptable. Some older men, or those with sexual anxiety, complain that its use may result in loss of erection. I consider this sometimes gives adequate grounds to prescribe a phosphodiesterase type-5 inhibitor (see BNF). For women who dislike the smell or messiness of semen, the condom solves their problem.

True rubber allergy can also occur (rarely), and can easily be solved by switching to a modern plastic condom.

Femidom

Femidom (Fig. 18) is a female condom comprising a polyurethane sac with an outer rim at the introitus and a loose inner ring, whose retaining action is similar to that of the rim of the diaphragm. It thus forms a well-lubricated secondary vagina. Available over the counter, along with a well-illustrated leaflet, it is completely resistant to damage by any chemicals with which it might come into contact. Using it, the penetrative phase of intercourse can feel more normal to the male partner and can also start before his erection is complete. However, couples should be forewarned to avoid the penis being wrongly positioned between the Femidom sac and the vaginal wall.

Reports about its acceptability are mixed, and a sense of humour certainly helps. There is evidence of a group of women (and their partners) who use it regularly, sometimes alternating with the male equivalent ('his' night then 'her' night). Others might also choose it, if it were more often mentioned by providers as even being an option. As the first female-controlled method with high potential for preventing HIV transmission, it must be welcomed.

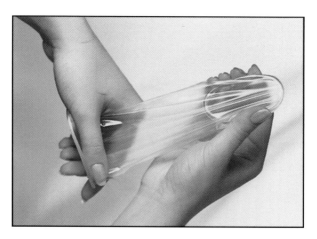

Figure 18
The female condom (Femidom). Source: Courtesy of Chartex International plc.

The cap or diaphragm

Though now considered 'old hat' and rarely used, many couples once initiated are pleasantly surprised at the simplicity of these vaginal barriers, although they are often acceptable only when sexual activity takes on a relatively regular pattern in a long-term relationship. They may be inserted well ahead of coitus, and so used without spoiling spontaneity. There is very little reduction in sexual sensitivity, as the clitoris and introitus are not affected.

Spermicide is recommended because no mechanical barrier is complete, although we still lack definitive research on this point.

Possible toxic effects of nonoxinol-9—which is unfortunately the only spermicidal agent marketed in the United Kingdom—to the vaginal wall have become a real concern (see below). However, the vagina is believed to be able to recover between applications when nonoxinol-9 is used in the manner, and at the kind of average coital frequency, of typical diaphragm-users.

The acceptability of the diaphragm itself depends on how it is offered. Its first-year failure rate, now estimated as high as 6 per 100 careful and consistent users, rising to 16 per 100 typical users (Table 1, p. 9) makes it *very unsuitable for most young women who would not accept pregnancy.* However, it suits others who are 'spacers' of their family. And it is capable of excellent protection above the age of 35 (3 per 100 woman-years, as the Oxford/FPA study reported in the early 1980s), provided it is as well taught and correctly and consistently used as it was by those couples.

FemCap^{TM} is since 2007 the only cervical cap on the UK market. Intended for provision through mainstream family planning clinics (supplier: Durbin), it is a useful alternative to the diaphragm, though in an RCT its 6-month failure rate was significantly higher, 13.5% compared with 7.9% for diaphragm users. It is a plastic cervical cap with a brim filling the fornices (displayed on right in Fig. 1, p .4) and comes in three sizes: so substituting for previously available cervical caps. It must be used with a spermicide but is reusable, with replacement recommended about every 2 years.

When there is great difficulty in inserting anything into the vagina—be it tampon, pessaries or a cap—the method is obviously not suitable. This problem may be connected with a psychosexual difficulty that may first present during the teaching of the method, but simple lack of anatomical knowledge is often involved.

Follow-up
Vaginal barriers should be checked initially after 1 to 2 weeks of trial, then annually. The fitting of diaphragms should be rechecked routinely post-partum, or if there is more than 3 kg gain or loss in weight.

If either partner returns complaining that they can feel any kind of cap during coitus, the fitting must be urgently checked. It could be too large or too small; or with the diaphragm the retro—pubic ledge may be insufficient to prevent the front slipping down the anterior vagina; or, most seriously, the item may be being placed regularly in the anterior fornix. The arcing spring diaphragm is then particularly useful.

Chronic cystitis may be exacerbated by pressure from a diaphragm's anterior rim. A smaller size may help. The condition was shown to occur less frequently with Femcap in the comparative pre-marketing trials.

For nurses or doctors who wish to offer this choice, there is no substitute for one-to-one training, both in the process of fitting the diaphragm and FemCap cervical cap and in teaching a woman how to use it correctly, backed by a good leaflet.

With these products, the single most important thing the woman must learn is the vital regular secondary check, after placing it, that she has covered her cervix correctly. A small group of usually older couples can and do use these methods successfully, but high motivation is essential. Once again, a good sense of humour helps.

Spermicides

Sadly, many useful products such as Delfen foam and the Today sponge have been removed from the UK market. At the time of writing (2012), the only spermicide available is Gygel™ contraceptive jelly with its applicator (shown in Fig. 1). This is now the only vaginal option in the United Kingdom for women of reduced fertility when a male or female condom or diaphragm or cap are unacceptable (see box).

Although invaluable as adjuncts to caps and diaphragms, used alone spermicides often fail since they do not reliably deal with a whole ejaculate. Yet spermicides can be used successfully by women whose natural fertility is reduced (see box below).

Gygel introduced via its applicator may be a satisfactory choice (though 100% effectiveness is never on offer):

- During full lactation as an alternative to the POP
- For women over 50 years of age for 1 year after periods cease (when contraception is still advised), whether or not they use HRT
- For women aged over 45 with secondary amenorrhoea (contraception being required for 2 years before menopausal infertility can be diagnosed)
- During continuing secondary amenorrhoea at a younger age, unless a COC is being used anyway to treat hypo-estrogenism
- As an adjunct to other contraception—e.g. spermicides may rarely be suggested as a supplement in couples who are not happy to stop using withdrawal as their main method—making it clear that the withdrawal must still continue. . . .

Many substances are well absorbed from the vagina, but there is no proof of systemic harm, congenital malformations or spontaneous abortions from the use of current spermicides, chiefly nonoxinol-9 or its close relatives.

Occasionally, sensitivity to a spermicide arises. More seriously, when used by Nairobi prostitutes four times a day for 14 days, nonoxinol-9 released from pessaries caused erythema and colposcopic evidence of minor damage to the vaginal skin.

Coupled with the doubts about its effectiveness against intracellular virus, it clearly should not be promoted as an anti-HIV virucide (see the systematic review by Wilkinson D, et al. Lancet Inf Dis 2002; 2:613–617). However, pending better alternatives, for the time being it remains good practice to continue to recommend nonoxinol-9 for normal contraceptive use (less frequently than four times a day!), whether alone or with diaphragms or FemCap, but not with condoms.

Final comment on spermicides

Worldwide, there remains a great unmet need for an effective user-friendly female-controlled vaginal microbicide, which might or might not also be a spermicide. Many international agencies are now actively involved, but progress is slow in this urgent and previously very neglected area of research.

FERTILITY AWARENESS AND METHODS FOR NATURAL REGULATION OF FERTILITY

At one time, these methods were generally despised and only adopted by those with strong religious views. Modern multiple index versions (based primarily on carefully charting changes to cervical mucus, the cervix itself by auto-palpation, and body temperature, with support from the so-called secondary indicators such as ovulation pain) are popular among those who prefer to use a more 'natural' method. There is no space here to do justice to this approach, but there is an extremely useful website which is secular and neutral in its approach: www.fertilityuk.org.

Those who wish to use these methods deserve careful explanation and ideally one-to-one teaching, particularly about charting the cyclical changes and the possible added use of other minor clinical indicators of fertility. Useful instruction leaflets, further advice and details of natural family planning (NFP) teachers (mostly non-NHS) available in different localities, can be obtained from www.fertilityuk.org (and also from the FPA website, www.fpa.org.uk). Additionally, they give advice about fertility awareness to *assist* conception.

With 'perfect use', the multiple index methods are capable of being acceptably effective. However, in the words of Professor Trussell of Princeton, they still remain 'very unforgiving of imperfect use'. Moreover, imperfect use is unfortunately common in the

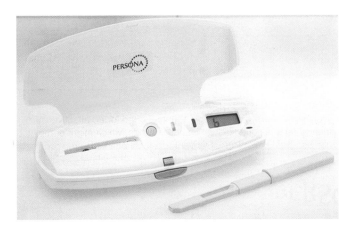

Figure 19
Persona. Source: Courtesy of Unipath Ltd.

real world. To be effective, many days of abstinence are inevitable and the highest possible cooperation from both parties is required but often lacking—especially from the male, whose motivation may well be suspect. (In one study, the failure rate was noted to be higher when the man rather than his partner was the one in charge of interpreting the temperature charts!) To be fair to the methods, failures also commonly result from poor use of other contraceptives, such as the condom, by those who do not wish to abstain during 'unsafe' days.

Persona™ (Unipath Ltd., Bedford, UK) (Fig. 19) is a combination of minilaboratory and microcomputer. It displays the 'safe' (green) and 'unsafe' (red) days of a woman's cycle, based on measurements of the first significant rise in her levels of urinary estrone-3-glucuronide and luteinizing hormone. With a reduced number of 'unsafe' days (8–10 for most women) being signalled per cycle, this contraceptive option is found by many couples to make things easier—but it does not apparently lead to greater effectiveness than careful charting of the indices with good compliance. The data on the failure rate are reported as 6 per 100 woman-years in the first year even with 'perfect use'—and Trussell (personal communication, 2003) still considers this to be an underestimate.

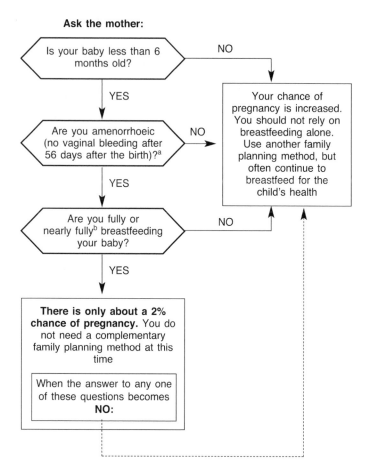

Ask the mother:

Is your baby less than 6 months old?

NO →

YES ↓

Are you amenorrhoeic (no vaginal bleeding after 56 days after the birth)?[a]

NO →

YES ↓

Are you fully or nearly fully[b] breastfeeding your baby?

NO →

YES ↓

Your chance of pregnancy is increased. You should not rely on breastfeeding alone. Use another family planning method, but often continue to breastfeed for the child's health

There is only about a 2% chance of pregnancy. You do not need a complementary family planning method at this time

When the answer to any one of these questions becomes **NO:**

[a]Spotting that occurs during the first 56 days is not considered to be menstruation.

[b]'Nearly' full breastfeeding means that the baby obtains almost 100% of its nutrition from the mother alone, and certainly no solid food.

Figure 20
Algorithm for the lactational amenorrhoea method (LAM).

Even on that slightly uncertain basis, couples should be informed that this is the same as a 1 in 17 risk of conceiving in the first year—on the high side, but perhaps good enough for 'spacers'.

For greater efficacy, couples should be advised:
- to use condoms on the pre-ovulatory days ('green days' if using Persona)—this being what I prefer to call the 'amber' phase (always less 'safe' because of the capriciousness of sperm survival in a woman)
- to abstain completely on all peri-ovulatory 'red days'
- to have unprotected intercourse only in the post-ovulatory phase—i.e. from the fourth day after 'peak mucus' or in the second green light phase with Persona

---

If Persona or another NFP method is to be commenced after any pregnancy or any hormone treatment—even just one course of hormonal EC—reliability demands that another method such as condoms or abstinence must first be used until there have been two normal cycles of an acceptable length (23–35 days).

Lactation within the specific guidelines of the lactational amenorrhoea method (LAM) as shown in Figure 20 constitutes a quintessentially 'natural method'—through to 6 months post-partum (see also p. 80).

Special considerations

HOW CAN A PROVIDER BE REASONABLY SURE THAT A WOMAN IS NOT PREGNANT, OR JUST ABOUT TO BE PREGNANT IN A CONCEPTION CYCLE?

UKMEC advises that the provider can be reasonably certain that the woman is not pregnant if she has no symptoms or signs of pregnancy and one or more of the following criteria apply:

1. She has not had intercourse since last normal menses.
2. She has been correctly and consistently using a reliable [sic] method of contraception.
3. She is within the first 7 days after (onset of) normal menses.
4. She is within 4 weeks post-partum for non-lactating women.
5. She is within the first 7 days post-abortion or miscarriage.
6. She is fully or nearly fully breastfeeding (as in LAM—Figure 20), amenorrhoeic and less than 6 months post-partum.

Note: Good clinical judgement is vital with respect to assessing the accuracy of the given history, including

- the absence of symptoms of pregnancy,
- the believability of reported abstinence,
- especially regarding point 2 in the list, the reliability of reported correct condom use is notoriously difficult to assess.

In the United Kingdom, these criteria can be reinforced by a urine pregnancy test with a sensitivity of at least 25 IU/L, but only if ≥3 weeks since the last UPSI. Such tests are not helpful if there could not possibly yet be an implanted blastocyst present—including, for example, at the time of most requests for EC with a normal last menstrual period (LMP).

SOME APPLICATIONS OF THE ABOVE
Quick starting

Traditionally 'medical' methods of contraception such as COCs have been scheduled always to start with or just after the woman's next menstrual period. This policy is now seen in many cases as having

- possibly been the cause of some avoidable conceptions and
- increased the chances that the woman never actually started her agreed new method in the next cycle.

Next-cycle commencement was devised mainly to avoid inadvertent use during early pregnancy. But that risk due to immediate commencement can be minimized; and moreover the risks to a fetus of short-term exposure to hormonal methods (other than co-cyprindiol and probably the LNG-IUS, see p. 140) are known to be small.

Quick starting means immediate starting of a medical method at first visit, late in the menstrual cycle or straight after EC. What follows is adapted from the very useful guidance of FSRH at www.fsrh.org/pdfs/CEUGuidanceQuickStartingContraception.pdf.

- If a health professional is reasonably sure that a woman is not pregnant or at risk of pregnancy (using one or more of the six criteria above), 'medical' contraception can be started immediately, i.e. quick started, *unless* the woman prefers to wait until her next period. Such practice is usually outside the product licence/device instructions (pp.173–5).
- If a health professional is reasonably sure that a woman is not pregnant or at risk of pregnancy from recent UPSI but her preferred contraceptive method is not available, combined hormonal contraception (CHC), the progestogen-only Pill (POP) or a progestogen-only injectable can be used as a *bridging method*. Though all of these are unlikely to be harmful if she conceives, women requesting the progestogen-only injectable (which cannot be rapidly discontinued) should ideally be offered one of the other bridging methods—Cerazette™ is often the best.

- When starting intrauterine methods or co-cyprindiol (Dianette®, Clairette®) health professionals should take particular care to exclude pregnancy, or risk of pregnancy from recent UPSI. If pregnancy cannot be excluded, the copper-bearing IUD may be started immediately if the criteria for use as EC are met. (Given fears re teratogenesis, insertion of the levonorgestrel-releasing IUS or initiation of co-cyprindiol should be delayed until pregnancy can be confidently excluded.)
- If pregnancy cannot be excluded (e.g. following administration of EC) but a woman is likely to continue to be at risk of pregnancy or has expressed a preference to start contraception without delay, immediate 'quick starting' of CHC or the POP or Cerazette may be considered. The woman should be informed of the potential risks and the need to have a pregnancy test at the appropriate time (see recommendation below).
- If contraception is quick started in **any** woman for whom the pregnancy risk is not nil, a (further) pregnancy test should be advised no sooner than 3 weeks from the last episode of UPSI.
- If starting hormonal contraception immediately after LNG-only EC, condoms or avoidance of sex should be advised for 7 days for CHCs (9 days for Qlaira®) and 2 days for POPs.
- If starting progestogen-containing hormonal contraception immediately after EC using the anti-progestogen ulipristal acetate, the FSRH recommends condoms or avoidance of sex for 7 days more than the usual time for each method (as in the last bullet): hence 14 days for CHCs (16 days for Qlaira) and 9 days if starting a POP (UULP). But immediate insertion of a copper IUD would usually be preferred here, especially if the coital history suggests implantation block is required.
- If in due course pregnancy is diagnosed after starting contraception and the woman wishes to continue with the pregnancy, the new method should usually be stopped or removed.

'Bridging'—a useful subset of quick starting

Bridging is a practice that can be *particularly helpful when dealing with uncertainty about the current conception risk, especially* in two common practical quandaries, in which the six WHO/UKMEC criteria above cannot be applied at the first visit. These women have regular UPSI, have secondary amenorrhoea and have no LMP, either because they are

- not breastfeeding and beyond 4 weeks post-partum (this being the time of first recorded ovulations), or
- more than 2 weeks overdue with DMPA injection, with the earliest UPSI also after the 14th week *and* more than 5 days ago so that hormonal EC is problematic (p. 152).

A pair of visits are needed, since a pre-diagnosable pregnancy (unimplanted blastocyst) might be present at the first.

First visit

Do a urine pregnancy test with sensitivity at least 25 IU/L. If this test is negative or not done, more assurance is required before, for example, inserting an LNG-IUS. She will probably laugh if you suggest the ideal, to abstain for a full 3 weeks since the most recent UPSI, so as to obtain a fully confirmatory negative pregnancy test. Instead, given that POPs have never been suspected of harming an early pregnancy, one of these may be prescribed until then as a bridging method: Cerazette often being chosen because of its efficacy (and rapid action, in 48-hours).

Second visit

When she returns, probably still amenorrhoeic, do a pregnancy test.
- If now she has no symptoms of pregnancy, plus the pregnancy test with sensitivity of ≤25 IU/L is negative, and
- the backup bridging method has reportedly been used well: insert the IUS or give the delayed dose of DMPA, and
- continue with the bridging method, discontinuing after 7 more days.

CONTRACEPTION FOR THE OLDER WOMAN
Maximum age for COC use

Smokers or others with arterial risk factors should always discontinue the CHC at age 35 (WHO 4)

But a **healthy, totally risk-factor-free woman (migraine-free, non-smoker),** provided with modern Pills and careful monitoring, may consider that the many gynaecological and other benefits of CHCs outweigh for her the small, though increasing, cardiovascular and breast cancer risks (p. 35 and p. 19) of the method up to age 50 to 51, which is the mean age of the menopause. Although there are usually better contraceptive choices—consider especially an intrauterine method—an appropriate CHC (usually the natural-estrogen-containing Qlaira or a 20-μg EE product) may therefore be used till then. For women with diminishing ovarian function but who need contraception as well, this is logical and may be preferable to standard hormone-replacement therapy (HRT) along with having to use some other contraceptive.

Beyond 50 to 51 years of age, the age-related increased COC risks are usually unacceptable for all, given that fertility is now so low that simple, virtually risk-free contraceptives will suffice.

Most forms of HRT are not contraceptive, but may be indicated combined with any simple contraceptive in symptomatic women when estrogen is no longer being supplied by the COC. Of course, the IUS-plus-HRT combination is a winner here, since it safely supplies contraceptive HRT with endometrial protection plus, usually, also highly acceptable oligo-amenorrhoea.

The actual and expected advantages of HRT by LNG-IUS (note: change at 4 years) plus estrogen by any route
- Contraceptive HRT
- No-period, usually no-bleed HRT—before proof of ovarian failure
- No heavy/painful loss HRT, or other menstrual symptoms
- Minimal systemic progestogen HRT
- Plus still giving the expected quality-of-life benefits of HRT

Diagnosing loss of fertility at the menopause

Although hormonal methods tend to mask the menopause, it is not always necessary to know the precise time of final ovarian failure. Unfortunately, follicle-stimulating hormone (FSH) levels are unreliable for diagnosis of complete loss of ovarian function. So one of the options in the boxes below should be followed.

> **Plan A Contraception may cease: after waiting for the 'officially approved' 1 year of amenorrhoea above age 50, having stopped all hormones**
> This is the obvious plan for
> - Copper IUDs*
> - Condoms
> - Gygel spermicide via applicator (which unlike in younger women may well suffice above age 50 when combined with amenorrhoea, though no-one can be promised 100% effectiveness)
>
> *IUDs (and IUSs) should be removed 1 year after the final bleed: if left in situ for many years post-menopausally, there have been case reports of severe actinomycosis.

But what to do if the woman is using one of the hormonal methods or HRT, which mask the menopause?

- If on DMPA or EE-containing COC (or other CHC): age 50 to 51 is the time to stop these. They are needlessly strong, contraceptively, and the known risks increase with age. Qlaira is a possible exception to this (see p. 69), usable if requested through to age 55 (see below).
- The POP, or an implant, or the LNG-IUS with or without HRT: as contraceptives these add negligible medical risks that increase with age—though the IUS should usually be removed no later than about 55 (actinomycosis risk, see box.)
- Therefore, one of these (usually the POP) may be continued until the latest age of potential fertility has been reached: then the woman just stops the contraception (no tests!). When is that?
  - A good estimate is age 55. The FSRH in its 2010 Guidance on contraception for women above 40 (see www.fsrh.org/pdfs/ContraceptionOver40July10.pdf) quotes Treloar's evidence that 95.9% have ceased menstruation forever by then (and such bleeds as may happen later, in the other 4.1%, would be unlikely to be related to cycles that were fertile).

Plan B Contraception may cease: at age 55, with no need for a confirmatory FSH level. This could be, for example, after having switched to or having continued till then with a progestogen-only method—most commonly a POP (old type)

- This appears an acceptably secure policy. It is true though that the *Guinness Book of Records* has reported some exceptionally rare cases of motherhood without medical intervention beyond age 55.
- As a safeguard, if (rarely) there still are (non-pathological) bleeding episodes after ceasing hormones at 55, the woman is advised to use a simple contraceptive such as vaginal spermicide or condoms and then report back later, when her periods appear to have finally ceased.

Plan C Contraception may cease: above age 50 if four criteria apply

Older users of hormonal contraception may cease using any method
IF:

1. They have passed their 50th birthday, **AND**, after a trial of 2 months' discontinuation using barriers or spermicides, they have:
2. Vasomotor symptoms
3. Two separate high FSH levels (>30 U/L) 1 month apart when off all treatment
4. Continuing amenorrhoea thereafter, beyond this trial period

With due warnings of lack of certainty, the FSRH agrees that these women may cease all contraception earlier than the approved 1 year post 50. Or, especially if bleeding episodes do return, simply use condoms or spermicide until there finally has been a full year of true amenorrhoea.

There are useful clues for COC-users and POP-users that discontinuation to follow the protocol in the above box is worth a try, namely:

- if COC-users start getting 'hot flushes' at the end of their Pill-free interval—especially if a high FSH result is obtained then.
- if old-type POP-users develop vasomotor symptoms with amenorrhoea (see p. 88).

Appendix

USE OF LICENSED PRODUCTS IN AN UNLICENSED WAY

Often, licensing procedures have not yet caught up with what is widely considered the best evidence-based practice. Such use is legitimate and may indeed be necessary for optimal contraceptive care, provided certain criteria are observed. These are well established (see FSRH Guidance, July 2005. J Fam Plann Reprod Health Care 2005; 31:225–242).

The prescribing physician must accept full liability and

- Adopt an evidence-based practice endorsed by a responsible body of professional opinion
- **Assess the individual's priorities and preferences,** giving a clear account of known and possible risks and benefits
- **Explain to her that it is an unlicensed prescription**
- **Obtain informed (verbal) consent and record this**
- Ensure good practice, including follow-up, to comply fully with professional indemnity requirements: along with meticulous record-keeping
- **Be prepared to provide, often, dedicated written materials:** because the manufacturer's PIL insert may not apply in one or more respects.

This protocol for unlicensed use of a licensed product is termed 'off-label' or sometimes **'named-patient' prescribing**.

Notes

1. Attention to the details is important—as in the (unlikely) event of a claim, the manufacturer can be excused from any liability if the prescription was not in line with the relevant SPC.

2. However, since the last edition of this book there has been one modification to the above protocol.

New GMC/FSRH/NMC advice (2008, 2009)

The third and fourth bullets above require a record that the woman understands and consents to this course of action, which though clearly evidence based, is not yet licensed. That practice remains medicolegally safe, and *indeed should continue unless* the particular unlicensed practice has become 'current practice' as described by the General Medical Council (GMC) in their document *Good Practice in Prescribing Medicines* (2008). Para 22 therein states that *'Where current practice supports the use of a medicine in this way it may not be necessary to draw attention to the licence when seeking consent'* (GMC: www.gmc-uk. org/static/documents/content/Good_Practice_in_Prescribing_Medicines_0911.pdf).

In 2009, the relevant committees of the FSRH agreed that the GMC's words: 'current practice supports the use' may be held to apply with respect to contraception if *'use falls within current guidance issued by the Faculty's Clinical Effectiveness Unit. Similarly, current guidance from the RCOG and NICE should be regarded as common practice'* www.fsrh.org/pdfs/JointStatementOffLabelPrescribing.pdf. In such instances, the slightly disturbing (for the woman) point about lack of licensing need not always be made and it may not be necessary for clinicians to document every occasion when a contraceptive preparation is prescribed outside the product licence. Current guidance to nurse/midwife prescribers is different.

The Nursing and Midwifery Council (NMC) advises that nurse or midwife independent prescribers may prescribe off-label if they are satisfied that this better serves the patient/client's needs, if they are satisfied that there is a sufficient evidence base and that they have explained to the patient/client the reasons why medicines are not licensed for their proposed use, and document accordingly. The NMC also states it is acceptable for medicines used outside the terms of the licence to be included in patient group directions (PGDs), when such use is justified by current best clinical practice and the direction clearly describes the status of the product.

EQUIVALENT PROPRIETARY NAMES FOR COMBINED PILLS WORLDWIDE

Until the fourth edition of this book, the above directory appeared in printed form. It listed details of the equivalent brand names used worldwide, identical with or very similar to currently marketed UK low-dose combined pills. The International Planned Parenthood Federation (IPPF) now has this directory in its entirety on its website (www.ippf.org). This now attempts to list the names of *all hormonal methods*, is accessible to all, is usually accurate, and regularly updated.

BELIEVABLE WEBSITES IN REPRODUCTIVE HEALTH

www.margaretpyke.org
Local services for London, contraceptive research—and superb training courses on offer

www.ippf.org
Online version of the Directory of Hormonal Contraception, giving equivalent pill brands used worldwide

www.who.int/reproductive-health
WHO's latest Eligibility criteria and new Practice recommendations

www.rcog.org.uk
Evidence-based College Guidelines on male and female sterilization, infertility and menorrhagia

www.fsrh.org
Website of Faculty of Sexual & Reproductive Health, includes Faculty Guidance pdfs on most methods, crucial topics such as Quick starting, access to the Journal of the Faculty, UK MEC—and more

www.nice.org.uk
Particularly useful for its LARC Guideline, others in reproductive health are anticipated

www.fpa.org.uk
Excellent helpline, 0845 122 8690. Patient information and essential leaflets! See also www.patient.co.uk

www.brook.org.uk
Similar to FPA website but for those <25; plus a really secure online enquiry service. Helpline 0800 0185023

www.fertilityuk.org
The fertility awareness and NFP service, including teachers available locally

www.bashh.org
National guidelines for the management of all STIs and a listing of GUM Clinics in the United Kingdom

www.gmc-uk.org/static/documents/content/0-18_0510.pdf

'0–18 years: guidance for all doctors'—gives ethical guidance on almost everything relevant to this group

www.ruthinking.co.uk equates to www.nhs.uk/Livewell/Sexandyoung-people; & www.likeitis.org/indexuk.html—SRH by/for the young

www.teenagehealthfreak.com
FAQs as asked by teens, on *all* health subjects, not just reproductive health—from Anorexia to Zits!

www.the-bms.org
Research-based advice on menopause and hormone-replacement therapy

www.familylives.org.uk (formerly parentline plus)
Top tips for parents regarding how to help their teens and preteens not to suffer many kinds of grief ...

www.relate.org.uk
Enter postcode to get nearest Relate centre for relationship counselling and psychosexual therapy

www.ipm.org.uk
Website of Institute of Psychosexual Medicine. Seminar training courses.

www.basrt.org.uk
Website of British Association for Sexual and Relationship Therapy. Provides a list of therapists

www.ecotimecapsule.com[1] & www.populationmatters.org[2] & www.populationandsustainability.org & www.willyoujoinus.com & www.peopleandplanet.net & www.popconnect.org (*for the Population Dots movie*)

(First two for John Guillebaud's 'Apology to the Future' project[1] and 'Youthquake' [2] = downloadable pdf)

FURTHER READING

Cooper E, Guillebaud J. Sexuality and Disability. London: Radcliffe Publishing, 1999.

Guillebaud J, MacGregor A. The Pill & Other Methods—the Facts. 7th ed. Oxford: OUP, 2009.

Guillebaud J, MacGregor A. Contraception—Your Questions Answered. 6th ed. Edinburgh: Elsevier (Churchill-Livingstone), 2012.

McVeigh E, Homburg R, Guillebaud J. Oxford Handbook of Reproductive Medicine and Family Planning. 2nd ed. Oxford: OUP, 2012.

Many more relevant book titles, as well as DVDs and useful patient leaflets concerning all methods, can be obtained by easy mail order from the UK Family Planning Association (fpa) and the International Planned Parenthood Federation (IPPF). See their websites above.

GLOSSARY

ALO	*Actinomyces*-like organisms
AMI	acute myocardial infarction
BBD	benign breast disease
BMD	bone mineral density
BMI	body mass index
BNF	British National Formulary
BP	blood pressure
BTB	breakthrough bleeding
CHC	combined hormonal contraception/ive
CIN	cervical intraepithelial neoplasia
COC	combined oral contraception/ive
COEC	combined oral emergency contraceptive
CPA	cyproterone acetate
CSM	Committee on the Safety of Medicines (UK)
CVS	cardiovascular system
DFFP	Diploma of the Faculty of Family Planning and Reproductive Health Care now the DFSRH
DFSRH	Diploma of the Faculty of Sexual and Reproductive Health
DM	diabetes mellitus
DMPA	depot medroxyprogesterone acetate (Depo-Provera)
DNA	deoxyribonucleic acid
DoH	Department of Health (now termed DH)
DSG	desogestrel
DSP	drospirenone
E2	estradiol
EC	emergency contraception
EE	ethinylestradiol
EVA	ethylene vinyl acetate

FSRH	Faculty of Sexual and Reproductive Health, formerly Faculty of Family Planning and Reproductive Health-care
FAQ	frequently asked question
FH	family history
fpa	family planning association
FSH	follicle-stimulating hormone
GMC	General Medical Council
GP	general practitioner
GSD	gestodene
GUM	genitourinary medicine
hCG	human chorionic gonadotrophin
HDL	high-density lipoprotein
HIV	human immunodeficiency virus
HMB	heavy menstrual bleeding
HPV	human papillomavirus
HRT	hormone replacement therapy
HUS	haemolytic uraemic syndrome
IPPF	International Planned Parenthood Federation
IUD	intrauterine device
IUS	intrauterine system
LAM	lactational amenorrhoea method
LARC	long-acting reversible contraceptive method
LCR	ligase chain reaction—ultrasensitive and specific test (e.g. for *Chlamydia*)
LMP	last menstrual period
LNG	levonorgestrel
LNG-IUS	Levonorgestrel-releasing intrauterine system
MFFP	Membership of the Faculty of Family Planning and Reproductive Health Care
MFSRH	Member(-ship) of the Faculty of Sexual & Reproductive Health
MHRA	Medicines and Healthcare Products Regulatory Agency
MPC	Margaret Pyke Centre
NET	norethisterone (termed norethindrone in the United States)
NETA	norethisterone acetate
NFP	natural family planning
NGM	norgestimate
NHS	National Health Service

NICE	National Institute for Health and Clinical Excellence
NMC	Nursing and Midwifery Council
OR	odds ratio
PCOS	polycystic ovarian syndrome
PCR	polymerase chain reaction (like LCR, for ultrasensitive/ specific tests)
PFI	pill-free interval
PGD	patient group directions
PID	pelvic inflammatory disease
PIL	patient information leaflet
PMDD	Premenstrual dysphoric disorder (US term for severe PMS)
PMS	premenstrual syndrome
POP	progestogen-only pill
RCGP	Royal College of General Practitioners
RCN	Royal College of Nursing
RCOG	Royal College of Obstetricians and Gynaecologists
RCT	randomized controlled trial
SHGB	sex-hormone-binding globulin
SLE	systemic lupus erythematosus
SPC	Summary of Product Characteristics (= Data Sheet)
SRE	sex and relationships education
SRH	Sexual and Reproductive Health
STI	sexually transmitted infection
TIA	transient ischaemic attack
TTP	thrombotic thrombocytopenic purpura
UKMEC	UK adaptation by the Faculty of SRH, of WHO's Medical Eligibility Criteria for contraceptive use
UPA	ulipristal acetate
URL	Uniform Resource Locator - on the internet
UPSI	unprotected sexual intercourse
VTE	venous thromboembolism
VV	varicose veins
WHO	World Health Organization
WHOMEC	WHO Medical Eligibility Criteria for contraceptive use
WHOSPR	WHO's Selected Practice Recommendations for contraceptive use

Index

Page numbers in italics indicate tables, boxes, or figures.